*Cross-Cultural Comparisons:
Data on Two Factors in Fertility Behavior*

RONALD FREEDMAN is a professor of sociology and associate director of the Population Studies Center, The University of Michigan, and LOLAGENE C. COOMBS is a research associate at the Population Studies Center.

Cross-Cultural Comparisons: Data on Two Factors in Fertility Behavior

REPORT OF A PROJECT OF THE SUBCOMMITTEE
ON COMPARATIVE FERTILITY ANALYSIS
OF THE INTERNATIONAL UNION
FOR THE SCIENTIFIC STUDY OF POPULATION

Prepared for the Subcommittee by:

Ronald Freedman, *Chairman*
Lolagene C. Coombs, *Coordinator*

AN OCCASIONAL PAPER OF THE POPULATION COUNCIL

The Population Council
245 Park Avenue
New York, New York 10017

The Population Council is an organization established in 1952 for scientific training and study in the field of population. It endeavors to advance knowledge in the broad field of population by fostering research, training, and technical consultation and assistance in the social and biomedical sciences.

The Council acknowledges, with thanks, the funds received from the Ford Foundation, the United Nations Fund for Population Activities, the United States Agency for International Development, the World Bank, and other donors for the publication program of the Population Council.

Copyright © 1974 by The Population Council
All rights reserved
Library of Congress Catalog Card Number: 74–80928
ISBN 0–87834–022–X
Printed in the United States of America

Distributed for The Population Council by
Key Book Service, Inc.
425 Asylum Street
Bridgeport, Connecticut 06610

CONTENTS

LIST OF TABLES ... ix

Introduction ... 1
Some General Methodological Problems ... 3
Participation and Support ... 5

ONE
Preferences about Sex of Children ... 9

Overview ... 11
Stated Preferences ... 12
Attitudinal Indicators ... 20
Behavioral Evidence ... 34
Conclusion ... 42

TWO
Practice of Contraception by Women Wanting No More Children ... 44

Overview ... 45
Variations with Wife's Age ... 47
Variations by Parity ... 55
Educational Differentials ... 59
On the Validity and Reliability of the Data ... 65

Appendix ONE
Summary Notes on Definitions   71

Appendix TWO
Methodological Statements for the Individual Studies   75

LIST OF TABLES

Table 1.1 Ideal Number of Sons: Percentage Distribution, for Married Women Aged 20–39 Years — 13

Table 1.2 Mean and Modal Number of Children and Sons Preferred, for Women Aged 20–39 Years, in Selected Populations — 14

Table 1.3 Ideal Number of Children: Percentage Distribution, for Married Women Aged 20–39 Years — 15

Table 1.4 Ideal Number of Sons: Percentage Distribution by Wife's Age and Ideal Number of Children, for Married Women Aged 20–39 Years — 16

Table 1.5 Modal Number of Sons Preferred by Women with Specified Ideal Number of Children, for Married Women Aged 20–39 Years — 19

Table 1.6 Mean Ideal Number of Sons, by Wife's Education and Urban-Rural Residence, for Married Women Aged 20–39 Years — 21

Table 1.7 Percentage Wanting No More Children and Mean Ideal Number of Children, for Women Aged 20–39 Years — 23

Table 1.8 Percentage Wanting No More Children by Number of Living Children and Sons, for Married Women Aged 20–39 Years — 24

Table 1.9 Inferences about Sex Preferences Based on Relationship of Parity and Sex Composition to Percentage Who Want No More Children; Number and Percent of Instances in Which Specified Relationship Holds—Data from Age Groups 20–29 and 30–39 — 28

Table 1.10 Mean Additional Number of Children Wanted, by Number of Living Children and Sons, for Married Women Aged 20–39 Years   30

Table 1.11 Percentage Who Expect More Than Ideal, by Number of Living Children and Sons, for Married Women Aged 20–39 Years   33

Table 1.12 Percentage Currently Using Contraception, by Number of Living Children and Sons, for Married Women Aged 20–39 Years   36

Table 1.13 Summary of Evidence for Sex Preference Based on Relationship of Parity and Sex Composition to Five Variables   38

Table 1.14 Parity Progression Ratios, by Wife's Age and Sex of Living Children, for Married Women Aged 20–39 Years Who Have Reached Specified Parities   40

Table 2.1 Ranges in Percents Wanting No More Children, Practicing Contraception, Not Practicing Contraception Among Those Who Want No More Children, and Not Practicing Contraception and Wanting No More Children, for Developed and Developing Countries, for Women Aged 30–39 Years   46

Table 2.2 Comparison of Selected Developed and Developing Countries with Respect to Percent Wanting No More Children, Practicing Contraception, Not Practicing Contraception Among Those Who Want No More Children, and Not Practicing Contraception and Wanting No More Children, for Women Aged 30–39 Years   46

Table 2.3 Percentage Wanting No More Children, by Wife's Age and Number of Living Children, for Married Women Aged 20–39 Years   48

Table 2.4 Percentage Currently Using Contraception, by Wife's Age and Number of Living Children, for Married Women Aged 20–39 Years   50

Table 2.5 Of Those Who Want No More Children, Percentage Not Using Contraception, by Wife's Age and Number of Living Children, for Married Women Aged 20–39 Years   52

Table 2.6 Percentage Who Want No More Children and Are Not Using Contraception, by Wife's Age and Number of Living Children, for Married Women Aged 20–39 Years 56

Table 2.7 Range in Percentage Wanting No More Children and Not Using Contraception, by Number of Living Children, for Developing and Developed Countries 58

Table 2.8 Percentage Wanting No More Children, by Wife's Age and Education, for Married Women Aged 20–39 Years 60

Table 2.9 Percentage Currently Using Contraception, by Wife's Age and Education, for Married Women Aged 20–39 Years 61

Table 2.10 Of Those Who Want No More Children, Percentage Not Using Contraception, by Wife's Age and Education, for Married Women Aged 20–39 Years 62

Table 2.11 Percentage Who Want No More Children and Are Not Using Contraception, by Wife's Age and Education, for Married Women Aged 20–39 Years 63

Table 2.12 Percentage Wanting No More Children and Contraceptive Status by Wife's Age and Education, for Married Women Aged 20–39 Years, for Four Developed Countries 66

Table 2.13 Trend for 1965–1970 in Attitudes About Number of Children and Use of Contraception, Taiwan, Married Women, Aged 30–39 Years 68

Introduction

This project was designed to investigate whether useful methodological and substantive findings can be derived from tabulations from different countries based on studies not originally planned in common for such a purpose. The idea evolved as one modest follow-up to a previous project of the International Union for the Scientific Study of Population (IUSSP) that developed a "model" questionnaire for fertility studies.[1] A more ambitious venture for international studies of comparable design has since been developed on a large scale by the World Fertility Survey, using newly developed model questionnaires. Closely coordinated projects have already been carried out in Latin America under the leadership of the Centro Latinoamericano de Demografía (CELADE); and the Economic Commission for Europe, through a Working Group on Social Demography, has organized a project for centrally processing and analyzing data from ten European countries, Turkey, and the United States.

The aim of this one-year IUSSP project was to focus the materials from a reasonable number of fertility surveys, carried out individually during the last decade, on a few specific questions, as the basis for a seminar conference and report. This publication stems from the report, and reveals not only the possibilities but some of the problems involved in this type of joint

---

[1] United Nations, *Variables and Questionnaire for Comparative Fertility Surveys*, Department of Economic and Social Affairs, Population Studies, no. 45 (New York: United Nations, 1970).

venture. The two specific substantive issues selected for comparative study were: (1) sex preference for children—its prevalence and relation to fertility behavior, and (2) wanting no more children but not practicing contraception—the prevalence and correlates of this phenomenon.

Ronald Freedman and Lolagene Coombs of the University of Michigan Population Studies Center organized and coordinated the IUSSP project, largely by mail. Because this was an exploratory investigation with limited objectives and limited budget with no paid central staff, worldwide coverage was not attempted. Initial contact was made with a number of investigators in Asian countries who were known to the organizers through their own work there to have done pertinent fertility surveys. This provided a range of cultural variation for developing countries and regions, for which the topics investigated have particular relevance. A number of European and American investigators were added to provide contrasts between developed and developing areas. African and Latin American investigators were not included because of the limitations of staff and resources.

Aside from the knowledge that the 17 participants were all competent investigators in the field, the organizers had little prior information on the coverage, quality, or comparability of specific data sets. Differences in questionnaires, concepts, modes and standards of field work, coding, and tabulation quickly became apparent as the data were assembled. They were not so great as might have been expected, however, because for some years the informal exchange of questionnaires and frequent reference to both the IUSSP model questionnaire manual and the KAP manual of the Population Council[2] had resulted in similar usages without any formal agreement by the researchers. The variations are set forth in Appendixes 1 and 2. The expected differences point up methodological questions; they also add to the complexity of the task of making substantive comparisons.

Some of the problems of detailed comparability could be resolved through considerable correspondence. Others would have required more face-to-face conferences or central tabulation of data. Aside from the fact that some countries[3] will not release primary data for tabulation elsewhere, limited time and funds precluded such an approach on this project. But, it should be clear that the essential aims of the joint project were to explore just such methodological problems as do emerge in trying to combine materials from separately collected and tabulated data, and to provide a partial

---

[2] *Selected Questionnaires on Knowledge, Attitudes and Practice of Family Planning* (New York: Population Council, 1967).

[3] Throughout this report the word "country" is often used for convenience, although the units represented in this analysis also include cities, areas, and regions.

answer to the question: Are broad comparisons possible, despite such differences?

The comparative tables and the substantive discussions presented here were not initially designed for publication, but were a vehicle for intensive seminar discussion of common problems by the 17 different investigators. The process was as important as the product. However, the participants thought that the resulting substantive data were sufficiently unique, especially for developing countries, to merit publication despite their limitations. The data also serve one of their original purposes: to point up methodological problems encountered in such an effort.

Some General Methodological Problems

The following specific methodological issues emerged as problems in the seminar discussion and in the analysis:

1. Not all of the variables are available for all studies, so some are necessarily omitted from some comparisons. Presumably, this problem could be avoided in a program like that of the World Fertility Survey with required common standards for questions, codes, and tabulations for all participants.

2. Apart from the problem of whether similar terms and categories have similar meanings, the widely differing distributions on such control characteristics as parity or education greatly complicate comparisons, especially between developed and developing countries. For example, for developing countries it is important to have categories distinguishing among those at the lower end of the educational scale where most of the population is concentrated; in developed countries the important distinctions are much higher in the educational scale. This problem might be solved by using a large number of categories to include both situations, but this was not possible in this study, given the limited sample sizes. In addition, there is the problem of whether, for example, "poor education" defined as "less than high school graduation" in one place and as "no education" in another are really equivalent. This is a general problem of all comparative studies.

3. In a number of the developing countries questions about ideal number of children or sons produced a significant number of indeterminate responses, for example, "up to God," "fate," or "don't know" or nonresponse. This problem was by no means general. In seven studies the proportion of indeterminate responses was less than 4 percent: Ankara, Calcutta, Delhi, Korea, Mexico City, the Philippines, and Taiwan.

In another five studies the number of indeterminate cases was larger but still a fairly small minority: West Malaysia, 1970—7 percent; West Malaysia, 1967—18 percent; urban Thailand—12 percent; rural Thailand —18 percent; India—26 percent.

In the two Indonesian studies the proportion of indeterminate responses was very large—49 percent in Jakarta and 71 percent in rural East Java. These two studies, based on limited fertility survey experience, did not use probes or give their interviewers specific training on this issue, as recommended in the IUSSP model questionnaire manual. Without further work, it is impossible to know whether the use of such procedures would have reduced the indeterminate responses substantially, with valid results, or whether the question about ideal number of children or sons really is not meaningful in the Indonesian context. Some suggestions for lines of further research on this problem are presented later.

In the substantive analyses, indeterminate cases were not assigned estimated values except for studies where they were so few (less than 2 percent) that estimation would not affect results. In all other cases, the means are based on determinate responses only. Assuming that those giving indeterminate responses might have a latent desire for larger numbers of children, mean values would be somewhat higher if they could be included, but only for India is it likely that the difference in the result would be substantial. The two Indonesian studies were not included in most tables involving ideal number of children or sons. In the few tables where the Indonesian ideal number of children data appear, the tabulation refers only to the minority responding.

4. Indeterminate responses on whether more children were wanted were less problematic than those on ideal number of children for two reasons. First, the number giving such responses was relatively small for all the countries for which we have reports.[4] Second, the procedure followed in computing the proportion wanting no more children makes it certain that the indeterminate responses did not inflate the statistic. In computing the proportion wanting no more children, all couples in each group, including the indeterminate cases, were included in the denominator. However, only couples who specifically said they wanted no more children were included in the numerator. Therefore, the proportions shown are conserva-

---

[4] The numbers of indeterminate cases were reported as follows: Ankara—2 percent; Calcutta—13 percent; Delhi—less than 1 percent; Korea—2 percent; Mexico City—2 percent; Taiwan, 1967 and 1970—less than 1 percent; rural Thailand—8 percent; urban Thailand—5 percent; West Malaysia, 1967—4 percent. The number indeterminate was not reported for the other developing populations.

tive, because we have implicitly grouped the indeterminate cases with those who wanted more children.

5. Quite apart from the problem of indeterminate responses, questions may be raised about the validity of the determinate answers. The seminar grappled with this problem and concluded that, while the problem was real and merited intensive study, there was no justification for rejecting out-of-hand the responses given by representative samples of the populations. Instead, the seminar agreed that further lines of work were desirable to better establish how valid and reliable such responses might be. The general issue and the suggested lines of work are discussed in more detail at the close of the substantive analyses. The issue is also discussed with specific reference to the Thailand data in an article published after the seminar by Knodel and Prachuabmoh.[5]

6. Measurement of attitudes about fertility emerged as a general problem in the seminar—for example, when it appeared that different measures of sex preference sometimes gave quite different results. The problem is that, as in many other areas of survey work, the investigators were using ad hoc measures, usually single questions whose reliability and validity were not established. There is a need for measures that use the answers to a set of questions that can be tested for internal coherence in scales or other logical frameworks. One by-product of the project has been the development and methodological testing by C. H. Coombs, G. McClelland, and L. C. Coombs of new, potentially more sensitive and powerful measures of preference for number and sex of children.[6]

Participation and Support

Most of the work for this project was contributed by the individual investigators and the project coordinators. A generous grant from the Swedish International Development Authority (SIDA) to the IUSSP covered the costs of the seminar conference held in Brussels and the costs of secretarial work and duplication of manuscripts and tables.

---

[5] J. Knodel and V. Prachuabmoh, "Desired family size in Thailand: Are the responses meaningful?" *Demography* 10, no. 4 (November 1973): 619–638.

[6] C. H. Coombs, G. H. McClelland, and L. C. Coombs, "The measurement and analysis of family composition preferences," *Michigan Mathematical Psychology Papers*, Report no. 73-5 (Ann Arbor: University of Michigan, 1973).

The following investigators participated in the project:

Name and Affiliation	Data Provided
Ramesh Chander Department of Statistics, Kuala Lumpur, Malaysia	West Malaysia, 1970
Mercedes Concepción The Population Institute, Manila, Philippines	Philippines
Bom Mo Chung The Korean Institute for Research in the Behavioral Sciences, Seoul, Korea	Korea
Lolagene Coombs Population Studies Center, University of Michigan, Ann Arbor, Michigan, USA	Subcommittee Coordinator; Taiwan
P. B. Desai Institute of Economic Growth, University of Delhi, India	Delhi
Ronald Freedman Population Studies Center, University of Michigan, Ann Arbor, Michigan, USA	Subcommittee Chairman; Taiwan
David Goldberg Population Studies Center, University of Michigan, Ann Arbor, Michigan, USA	Ankara, Turkey; Mexico City
H. J. Heeren Institute of Sociology, Utrecht State University, Utrecht, The Netherlands	The Netherlands
N. Iskandar Institute of Demography, University of Indonesia, Jakarta, Indonesia	Jakarta
Andras Klinger Demographic Division, Hungarian Central Statistical Office, Budapest, Hungary	Hungary

Name and Affiliation	Data Provided
Christopher Langford Population Investigation Committee, London School of Economics, London, UK	Great Britain
Jean Morsa Free University of Brussels, Brussels, Belgium	Belgium
James Palmore East-West Center, University of Hawaii, Honolulu, Hawaii	West Malaysia, 1966–1967; Korea
R. H. Pardoko National Institute of Public Health, Surabaya, Indonesia	East Java
Visid Prachuabmoh Institute of Population Studies, Chulalongkorn University, Bangkok, Thailand	Thailand
M. V. Raman Indian Statistical Institute, Calcutta, India	Calcutta
D. V. N. Sarma Operations Research Group, Baroda, India and Anrudh Jain Population Council, New Delhi, India	India
T. H. Sun Taiwan Provincial Committee on Family Planning, Taichung, Taiwan	Taiwan
Charles Westoff and Ronald Rindfuss Office of Population Research, Princeton University, Princeton, New Jersey, USA	United States

The substantive sections and the related tables that follow were prepared for the Subcommittee by Lolagene C. Coombs and Ronald Freedman, both of the University of Michigan Population Studies Center. The initial versions of these substantive statements were reviewed by all participating investigators. Some changes had to be made without such consultation in the final editorial process before publication. Lolagene Coombs assumed principal responsibility for the section on sex preference; Ronald Freedman assumed principal responsibility for the section about those wanting no more children but not using contraception.

ONE

Preferences about Sex of Children

The question of the existence of preferences about the sex of children is important for demographers because of the possible influence of such preferences on the process of family formation and on completed family size. Couples with a strong preference for one sex, or for at least one child of each sex, may go beyond their desired family size in the event that they do not achieve the sex composition they want by the time their preferred number of children is reached. Mindel Sheps has shown mathematically that if the probability of having a boy is the same for all individuals, a sex preference will not affect the sex ratio in the population, but the expected family size will increase with increasing preference for one sex over the other.[1] There may be a conflict between a strong sex preference and a preference for a small family, and in that case there is a question of which will dominate. But if a couple's sex preference is not satisfied by the time their desired small size family is achieved, their motivation to practice contraception effectively may be lower and they may have more children than they originally intended, in the hopes of having a child of the desired sex.

In developed countries, sex preferences have been considered so unimportant recently that data on this issue are rarely collected in fertility studies. It is, however, often assumed that in most developing countries, a preference for sons, resulting from family values that emphasize the im-

---

[1] Mindel C. Sheps, "Effects on family size and sex ratio of preferences regarding the sex of children," *Population Studies* 17 (1963): 66–72.

portance of sons for economic, lineage, or religious reasons, is not only widespread but also rather uniformly exhibited, and that it is an important factor in fertility.

The comparative data assembled in this study indicate that, although there are divergences between the developing and the more developed countries in son preference, there is also considerable variation among the developing countries.

Inferences about the extent of sex preference and its influence on fertility behavior depend in part on the variables used to index such preference. At the outset of this comparative analysis project, it was recognized that on the basis of data collected, there was no adequate direct measure of sex preference, no single index that could be used comparably across cultures. Further, it was found that the statistic on number of sons wanted or considered ideal was of little value as an indicator of sex preference unless viewed in combination with the total number of children considered ideal. There was no unambiguous method for disentangling a preference for sex of child from preference for a given number of children. These are serious measurement problems, and one of the by-products of this project has been the development of new and potentially more powerful measures of preference for both number and sex of children.[2] Nevertheless, in the absence of such measures, it is still possible to use a number of plausible, if imperfect, indicators of sex preference, for which there are data for many of the populations considered in this study. The specific variables used here are:

1. Stated preferences, about desired or ideal number of children and sons.
2. Attitudinal indicators—attitudes and expectations about further childbearing, for women with a given number and sex of children, namely: percent who want no more children; mean additional children wanted; and percent who expect to have more children than they consider ideal.
3. Behavioral indicators—present and past behavior, for women with a given number and sex of children, namely: percent currently practicing contraception; parity progression ratios—the percent at parity x who go on to have $x + 1$ children.[3]

---

[2] See C. H. Coombs, G. H. McClelland, and L. C. Coombs, "The measurement and analysis of family composition preferences," *Michigan Mathematical Psychology Papers*, Report no. 73-5 (Ann Arbor: University of Michigan, 1973).

[3] The variables listed under 2 and 3 may be viewed as a set of conditional probabilities

Overview

Before presenting the detailed discussion of the data and the study variations, a brief overview may be useful. Inferences about the prevalence of sex-preference patterns in particular countries vary somewhat with the measure used. Differences in the character of the data (definitions, coding, and tabulations)[4] also may affect some comparisons. Nevertheless, it is feasible, based on the evidence discussed later in this report, to tentatively group countries, regions, and cities into three broad sets.

Group I: Those with a son preference. Included in this group are Korea, Taiwan, and India and Delhi on most variables. On some variables this group would also include Ankara and Mexico City.

Group II: An intermediate group, with no consistent preference pattern in the variables considered. Included are Calcutta, Jakarta, the Philippines, rural East Java, Thailand,[5] and probably West Malaysia.

Group III: Those showing no son preference, but with some evidence of a preference for at least one child of each sex. Countries in this group are Belgium, Great Britain, Hungary, and the United States.

These groupings obviously are not rigid, particularly because different measures yield somewhat different inferences. The exact grouping is not important, based as it must be on certain arbitrary ground rules discussed later. The fact of the wide range in evidence of sex preference is the relevant issue. The populations in both Group I and Group II are considered to be among the developing countries; however, the attitudes and behavior

---

of holding certain views or exhibiting specific behavior, depending on family composition at a selected parity and at a given point in time. While all these variables can be thought of as conditional probabilities, most differ from the parity progression ratios in that we can make inferences from attitude and behavior only at one point in time, that of the interview date. If we had data about attitudes and use of contraception at each parity a woman has ever reached, however, we could obtain (in a table similar to the parity progression ratios) the conditional probabilities of, for example, wanting no more children or using contraception, depending on the sex composition of the family at any given stage of the family building cycle.

[4] See Introduction and Appendixes 1 and 2 for a discussion of variations.

[5] Later analysis of data for Thailand shows that by the criteria used here sex preference appears to be fairly strong for the Chinese ethnic minority but not for other Thais. See John Knodel and Visid Prachuabmoh, "Desired family size in Thailand: Are the responses meaningful?" *Demography* 10, no. 4 (November 1973): 619–638. West Malaysia may show similar ethnic differences in sex preference.

are not uniform in regard to son preference. Such a preference appears more consistently in some developing countries than in others. The western populations in Group III, however, are clearly quite divergent from the developing populations in preferences as to number and sex of children and are reasonably similar to each other. By almost every criterion used, sex preference does not appear to be very important in any of the developed countries considered.

The parities[6] at which the preferences and attitudes may make an appreciable difference in behavior vary with the culture. In a culture with small family size norms, the critical parity may be the second, although the pressure for a small number of children may dominate any preference for sex of child, and the indicators used here may not reflect any sex preference that might really exist. If the ideal family size is larger, sex preference may not affect behavior until later in the family cycle, perhaps at third or fourth parity. If the ideal size is very large, so that most women who can do so go on to have as many as five children, then sex preferences may be less important in their impact because the probability of satisfying a preference for a particular sex is much greater if there are more children. If the desired number of children is moderate and there is a preference for sons, then the effects on population growth may be considerable. This situation is characteristic of some of the developing areas where family size values apparently center on having a moderate number of children, such as three or four. As modernization proceeds, some countries in which preference for larger families is now widespread will probably reduce size preferences. If this occurs without a corresponding decrease in the preference for sons, the son preference would influence fertility decisions even more often, since fewer couples would have the number of sons they want simply by chance as would be the case with larger numbers of children.

Stated Preferences

Stated preferences for sex of children (personal ideal) vary considerably, both within and among populations. Even in European countries where the mean desired family size is low, individual preferences range from none to as many as four or more sons (see Table 1.1). In Hungary, for example,

---

[6] For simplicity in discussion, the word "parity" is used frequently in place of "number of living children." The latter is the independent variable used throughout except for data from Great Britain, which are based on number of children ever born.

Table 1.1 Ideal Number of Sons: Percentage Distribution, for Married Women Aged 20–39 Years

Country, city, or region	Ideal number of sons							Number of cases	Mean ideal number of sons
	0	1	2	3	4 or more	boy or girl	Indeterminate		
Calcutta, 1970	0	32	57	9	2	*	0	947	1.8
Delhi, 1968–69	0	31	63	5	1	*	1	5,242	1.8
India, 1970	4	25	39	19	13	*	*	10,246	2.2
Rural East Java, 1972	1	7	15	5	1	*	71	1,418	2.1
Jakarta, 1968	1	7	22	17	3	5	46	811	2.4
Korea, 1971	0	6	67	24	1	1	1	1,620	2.2
West Malaysia, 1966–67	0	9	28	20	12	11	20	4,242	2.5
West Malaysia, 1970	1	11	44	23	9	4	7	13,449	2.4
Philippines, 1968	1	10	36	30	21	*	3	28,632[a]	2.7
Taiwan, 1967	0	8	68	18	2	2	1	4,300	2.1
Belgium, 1966	13	46	20	3	0	5	12	2,566	1.2
Hungary, 1966	21	56	19	3	1	*	*	5,208	1.0
United States, 1970	3	53	36	4	1	*	3	4,685	1.5

NOTE: See Appendix 1, item 1 for definitions.

* = No such category.

[a] Frequency is weighted as follows: urban respondents × 4 and rural respondents × 12.

whereas 21 percent of respondents want no sons, 1 percent want four or more sons.[7] The modal preference is one son. West Malaysia in 1966–1967 presents another extreme: less than 1 percent want no sons; 12 percent prefer four or more; and 31 percent respond that either a boy or a girl is all right or are indeterminate on the question.[8]

---

[7] For the sake of simplicity, most of the comparative material presented is based on the total age group 20–39 years. For the most part the patterns observed are similar for the younger and the older women, although the level of occurrence of a particular phenomenon is usually different.

[8] Data for West Malaysia are for two time periods. Reference to West Malaysia with no date means that the statement is accurate for both the 1966–1967 and the 1970 surveys. Where a comment applies to, or information is known for, only one of the studies, the date is given. There are also data for two time periods for United States (1965 and 1970), where data for some variables are available for one date or the other, and for Taiwan (1967 and 1970). No trend analysis is undertaken here; however, West Malaysian data for the two time periods are shown for some variables because there has been a marked increase in the use of contraception.

Table 1.2 Mean and Modal Number of Children and Sons Preferred, for Women Aged 20–39 Years, in Selected Populations

Country, city, or region	Mean number children[a]	Mean number sons	Modal number children	Modal number sons
India	3.7	2.2	3(4)[b]	2
Calcutta	3.0	1.8	3	2
Korea	3.7	2.2	3(4)	2
Taiwan, 1967	3.9	2.1	4	2
West Malaysia, 1966–67	4.8	2.5	5+	2(3+)
Philippines	*	2.7	*	2(3)
Belgium	2.6	1.2	2	1
Hungary	2.2	1.0	2	1
United States, 1970	2.8	1.5	2(3)	1

NOTE: See Appendix 1, items 1 and 2 for definitions.
* = No data.
[a] Except for Calcutta and Taiwan means on number of children preferred are calculated from the tabulated distributions: "0 and 1" counted as 1, "5 or more" counted as 6, "indeterminate" excluded.
[b] Indicates that at least 25 percent of the cases preferred the number in parentheses.

The populations for which we have data on ideal number of sons fall into two groups: those with a modal preference for two sons (including India, Calcutta, Delhi, rural East Java, Jakarta, Korea, West Malaysia, the Philippines, and Taiwan), and those with a modal preference for one son (Belgium, Hungary, and the United States). Obviously, wanting two sons rather than one does not necessarily mean a preference for boys rather than girls, since it is possible to prefer relatively large numbers of both sexes. Those areas with a greater preference for a higher number of sons also have a higher preferred number of children, but the relation of sons to total number of children wanted is not the same for all (see Table 1.2). Ideal number of children ranges widely as does ideal number of sons. In Taiwan (Table 1.3), to cite a developing population, almost no one wants one child, while 63 percent want four or more. In Belgium, the corresponding figures are 12 percent wanting one child and 18 percent wanting four or more.

Relation to Number of Children Preferred

Comparisons made on the basis of only the number of sons preferred may be quite misleading. For example, two women may each prefer to have two sons. But if one wants two children (and wants both to be sons) and the

Table 1.3 Ideal Number of Children: Percentage Distribution, for Married Women Aged 20–39 Years

Country, city, or region	Ideal number of children						Number of cases	Mean ideal number of children[a]
	1	2	3	4	5 or more	Indeterminate		
Ankara, 1966[b]	5	40	29	14	12	*	552	3.0
Calcutta, 1970	1	31	41	23	4	0	947	3.0
Delhi, 1968–69[b]	1	31	48	18	2	0	5,242	2.9
India, 1970[c]	0	8	30	23	12	26	10,246	3.7
Rural East Java, 1972	0	3	6	12	8	71	1,418	4.2
Jakarta, 1968	0	3	5	17	27	49	811	4.9
Korea, 1971	0	6	50	25	19	*	1,612	3.7
West Malaysia, 1966–67	0	5	10	21	46	18	4,242	4.4
West Malaysia, 1970	1	8	12	34	38	7	13,449	4.5
Mexico City, 1971[b]	2	14	20	35	28	*	486	4.0
Taiwan, 1967	0	7	28	46	17	1	4,300	3.9
Thailand (urban), 1970[c]	1	19	20	30	18	12	1,063	3.3
Thailand (rural), 1969[c]	3	15	17	20	27	18	639	4.0
Belgium, 1966[b]	12	43	21	14	4	7	2,566	2.6
Great Britain, 1967–68[b]	4	48	22	15	4	6	1,088	2.7
Hungary, 1966[b]	11	64	16	3	1	5	5,937	2.2
United States, 1970	2	49	23	21	5	1	4,684	2.8

NOTE: See Appendix 1, item 2 for definitions.
* = No such category.
[a] Except for Calcutta, West Malaysia, and Taiwan, means are calculated from the distributions: "0 and 1" counted as 1, "5 or more" counted as 6, "indeterminate" excluded.
[b] "0 and 1 children" combined as "1."
[c] "Indeterminate" and "no answer" combined as "indeterminate."

other wants four or five, we cannot assume that the degree of sex preference for the two women is the same. Preference for a specific number of sons is related to preference for total size of family, and it is only when we examine them in combination that evidence for the preference for sons can emerge (see Table 1.4). Variations in definition affect somewhat the interpretations that would be made for the individual population, but it is doubtful that they affect the broad patterns that emerge when countries are compared.[9]

---

[9] See Appendix 1 for details on definition variations.

Table 1.4 Ideal Number of Sons: Percentage Distribution by Wife's Age and Ideal Number of Children, for Married Women Aged 20–39 Years

Wife's age (years) and ideal number of children	Calcutta 1970				Delhi 1968-69				India 1970				Rural East Java 1972				Jakarta 1968				Korea 1971			
	≤1	2	3	4+	≤1	2	3	4+	≤1	2	3	4+	≤1	2	3	4+	≤1	2	3	4+	≤1	2	3	4+
20–29																								
1 child	36	56	7	2	35	59	4	0	31	42	16	10	10	19	6	0	7	25	16	3	9	73	15	1
2	99	1	0	0	—	—	—	—	91	2	7	0	—	—	—	—	—	—	—	—	91	5	0	0
3	2	98	0	0	96	3	0	0	64	30	3	2	96	4	0	0	—	—	—	—	0	98	0	0
4	0	73	27	0	1	98	0	0	34	50	12	4	47	51	2	0	7	84	9	0	0	74	24	1
5	—	—	—	—	0	82	17	0	22	50	19	9	10	83	7	0	4	47	47	0	0	2	91	3
6 or more	*	*	*	*	0	5	84	11	15	28	34	23	7	42	46	5	2	7	63	21	—	—	—	—
30–39																								
1 child	29	59	10	2	27	66	6	1	26	36	21	16	5	11	5	2	7	20	17	4	4	63	30	2
2	98	2	0	0	—	—	—	—	48	5	47	0	—	—	—	—	—	—	—	—	84	14	0	0
3	2	98	0	0	96	2	0	0	58	27	7	8	56	44	0	0	—	—	—	—	1	96	2	0
4	0	70	30	0	1	98	0	0	26	44	18	11	8	86	5	2	7	87	2	2	0	74	26	1
5	0	0	54	46	4	7	74	14	22	35	27	15	14	35	46	5	0	33	54	4	0	0	98	1
6 or more	*	*	*	*	0	8	33	58	13	33	30	24	7	11	52	30	0	7	66	23	0	0	50	50
20–39																								
1 child	32	57	9	2	31	63	5	1	29	39	19	13	8	15	5	1	7	22	17	3	6	67	24	1
2	98	2	0	0	65	0	0	0	82	2	16	0	—	—	—	—	—	—	—	—	87	10	0	0
3	2	98	0	0	96	3	0	0	61	29	5	5	98	2	0	0	62	14	0	0	1	97	1	0
4	0	72	28	0	0	82	17	0	31	47	15	7	50	49	1	0	68	27	0	0	0	74	25	1
5	3	0	50	47	2	6	78	13	22	43	23	12	9	84	6	1	7	85	6	1	0	1	96	2
6 or more	*	*	*	*	0	6	35	59	8	22	33	37	10	38	46	5	2	40	50	2	0	0	52	39
Number of Cases	947				5,242				10,246				1,418				811				1,614			

NOTE: See Appendix 1, items 1 and 2 for definitions. Distributions do not add to 100 percent because the categories "boy or girl" and "indeterminate" are omitted.

— = Less than 20 cases in the category.
* = No such category.

Table 1.4 (Continued)

Wife's age (years) and ideal number of children	West Malaysia 1966-67					West Malaysia 1970					Taiwan 1967					Belgium 1966					Hungary 1966					United States 1970				
	≤1	2	3	4+		≤1	2	3	4+		≤1	2	3	4+		0	1	2	3+		0	1	2	3+		0	1	2	3+	
20–29	11	32	20	11		14	50	21	6		10	73	12	1		15	50	18	2		18	66	14	2		2	57	34	4	
1 child	—	—	—	—		86	0	0	0		—	—	—	—		59	34	0	0		49	51	0	0		30	57	0	0	
2	89	8	0	0		94	4	0	0		78	15	0	0		8	82	5	0		11	77	12	0		2	93	4	0	
3	25	53	5	0		22	67	2	0		4	89	3	0		5	43	33	2		10	40	45	5		2	28	64	3	
4	6	70	12	1		2	90	5	0		1	88	9	0		2	2	82	6		5	32	40	23		1	2	92	3	
5	2	37	45	4		2	27	63	4		1	15	75	7		—	—	—	—		—	—	—	—		0	3	32	63	
6 or more	1	7	34	42		1	6	54	35		0	11	74	15		—	—	—	—		—	—	—	—		2	2	7	86	
30–39	8	25	19	13		10	39	25	12		6	64	24	4		12	44	21	4		22	50	22	6		3	48	39	6	
1 child	—	—	—	—		91	0	0	0		—	—	—	—		58	27	0	0		46	50	4	0		55	45	0	0	
2	79	4	0	0		90	5	0	0		87	10	0	0		10	79	4	0		18	60	22	1		2	89	5	0	
3	28	50	1	0		23	66	2	0		4	90	4	0		3	42	29	3		11	36	42	10		3	31	57	5	
4	6	73	8	0		2	87	7	0		2	84	13	0		2	6	80	5		2	24	37	36		1	1	92	5	
5	7	25	45	4		2	24	64	6		3	13	76	8		2	4	40	30		2	12	23	62		0	3	38	59	
6 or more	0	7	32	37		1	7	45	42		2	9	57	30		0	0	8	65		0	3	13	84		0	2	6	88	
20–39	9	28	20	12		12	44	23	9		8	68	18	2		13	46	20	3		21	56	19	4		3	53	36	5	
1 child	70	0	0	0		89	0	0	0		—	—	—	—		58	30	0	0		47	50	3	0		42	52	0	0	
2	85	7	0	0		92	4	0	0		81	13	0	0		9	80	4	0		15	68	17	1		2	91	5	0	
3	26	52	3	0		23	67	2	0		4	90	3	0		4	42	30	2		11	38	43	8		3	29	61	4	
4	6	71	10	1		2	89	6	0		1	86	11	0		2	5	80	5		3	26	38	33		1	1	92	4	
5	4	31	45	4		2	25	63	5		2	14	76	7		1	3	40	29		3	14	25	57		0	3	36	61	
6 or more	0	7	33	39		1	7	48	39		2	10	61	26		0	0	9	66		0	5	12	84		1	2	7	87	
Number of Cases	4,242					13,449					4,300					2,467					5,155					4,684				

If we consider the most frequently preferred number of sons among respondents with specified ideal number of children, the patterns exhibited in the developing areas vary somewhat, but as a whole are quite different from those in the developed countries. The developing and developed countries differ least when the desired number of children is an even number—two or four. In all areas, the modal preference for those with an ideal of two children is one son; for those with an ideal of four children the modal preference is two sons.[10] Thus, with an even number, where balance in sex composition is possible, the general preference in these data is for balance. When the ideal is four, however, in some of the developing areas, such as Korea, a considerable proportion (at least 25 percent) prefer three rather than two sons, whereas in the western countries the second most frequent preference is for fewer sons[11] (see Table 1.5). In every developing population, among those with an ideal of four children, the proportion who choose three or four sons is greater than the proportion who choose three or four daughters. We may speculate that in countries with higher ideal family size, one reason for wanting three or four children may be to increase the probability of getting the number of sons preferred.

When an odd number of children is preferred, and the number of boys and girls cannot be equal, in most developing countries a high proportion of women chose two boys for the three-child family and three boys for the five-child family, although the percentage making such choices varies considerably. In developed countries the situation is less consistent. When the ideal is three children, in Belgium the modal number of boys preferred is one, with the next most frequent preference being two. In Hungary and the United States, the modal preference is for two sons, although a considerable minority of respondents choose one. The number of respondents in developed countries who prefer either as few children as one or as many as five is small, and among these there is no consistent pattern of sex preference. Overall, this group of developed countries, in contrast to the developing countries, does not evidence any consistent preference for sons (see Tables 1.4 and 1.5).

---

[10] Because of the large number of indeterminate cases in the Jakarta and rural East Java studies, those studies should probably be excluded from this general statement, although it does hold for those respondents who gave specific answers.

[11] The numbers in brackets in Table 1.5 indicate the number of sons that at least 25 percent of the cases prefer—the number next highest in frequency to the modal number. In Calcutta, for example, among women whose ideal is four children, the modal choice for 72 percent of the cases is two sons. But 28 percent prefer three sons, indicating a moderate leaning toward a higher son preference. (Percentages come from Table 1.4.)

Table 1.5 Modal Number of Sons Preferred by Women with Specified Ideal Number of Children, for Married Women Aged 20–39 Years

Country, city, or region	Modal number of sons preferred if ideal number of children is:						Number of cases
	1	2	3	4	5	6+	
Calcutta, 1970	— (1)[a]	1 (34)	2 (42)	2[3][b] (20)	3 (3)	— *	947
Delhi, 1968–69	1 (1)	1 (31)	2 (48)	2 (18)	3 (2)	4+[3] (1)	5,242
India, 1970	1 (0)	1[2] (8)	2[1] (30)	2 (23)	3[2] (7)	4+[3] (3)	10,246
Rural East Java, 1972	— (0)	1 (3)	1,2 (6)	2 (12)	3 (6)	3 (3)	1,418
Jakarta, 1968	1 (0)	1 (3)	1[2] (5)	2 (17)	3[2] (13)	3 (14)	811
Korea, 1971	— (0)	1 (6)	2 (50)	2[3] (25)	3 (16)	3[4+] (2)	1,614
West Malaysia, 1966–67	1 (0)	1 (5)	2[1] (10)	2 (21)	3[2] (18)	4+[3] (28)	4,242
Taiwan, 1967	— (0)	1 (7)	2 (28)	2 (46)	3 (12)	3[4+] (5)	4,300
Belgium, 1966	0[1] (12)	1 (43)	1[2] (21)	2 (14)	2[3] (2)	3 (2)	2,567
Hungary, 1966	1[0] (14)	1 (68)	2[1] (12)	2[1,3+] (2)	3[2] (1)	3 (0)	5,937
United States, 1970	1[0] (1)	1 (49)	2[1] (23)	2 (21)	3[2] (2)	3 (2)	4,684

NOTE: See Appendix 1, items 1 and 2 for definitions.
— = Less than 20 cases preferring x number of children.
* = No such category.
[a] Percent with x ideal number of children, indicating relative importance of such choices for the population as a whole in a particular area. Percentages do not total 100 because indeterminates are not shown here; see Table 1.1.
[b] Indicates that at least 25 percent of the cases prefer number of sons indicated in the brackets.

Although there is evidence from these data of a fairly strong, though somewhat varied, preference for sons in some developing countries, in no country is there evidence of a wish to have no girls at all. However, of all the populations included in this analysis, Belgium is the only one that, on the basis of these variables, could be considered as having a slight preference for girls, although certainly not to the exclusion of boys.

Educational and Urban/Rural Differentials

In the developing countries, the preferred number of sons and the preferred number of children are somewhat greater among the less educated and more rural segments of the population (see Table 1.6).[12] For example, in Calcutta, women in the lowest educational category prefer 3.4 children and 2.1 sons, those in the highest category prefer 2.4 children and 1.4 sons. In Taiwan, although a large majority in all educational strata prefer three or four children and two sons, a significant minority (20 percent) of the better educated wants only two children and one son, and a similar minority of the more poorly educated wants five or more children and three or more sons. Among the less educated and more rural, the desire for a larger family may be a reflection of the desire for more sons.

In contrast, in the European countries there is little difference in either sex or number preference among the various educational or urban-rural strata. A modal preference for two children and one son appears in both Belgium and Hungary in all major strata. The United States shows more variation: women with junior high school or less education have a mean ideal of 3.7 children and 1.7 sons, while those with senior high or more education consider 2.9 children and 1.4 sons ideal.

Education and, to a lesser degree, urbanization seem to be factors in the value placed on sons, but any definitive separation of their effects would require more detailed tabulations (difficult with the number of cases in most studies), or a multivariate statistical analysis, which was not feasible for many of the investigators in this study.

The stated preferences considered so far are useful descriptively, but are not very satisfactory measures of sex preference. Preferences for number and for sex of children must be considered jointly in these data and cross-cultural comparisons are cumbersome and difficult. However, if sex preferences do exist, we would expect them to be reflected in respondents' attitudes about future childbearing and to affect behavior. Data for a number of variables from which inferences about sex preference may be made are discussed in the following sections.

Attitudinal Indicators

Preference for children of a particular sex may be inferred from attitudes toward having more children. Although some sex preferences may not

---

[12] Mean ideal number of children by education was not specified in the initial tabulation plan but was supplied by a few researchers.

Table 1.6 Mean Ideal Number of Sons, by Wife's Education and Urban-Rural Residence, for Married Women Aged 20–39 Years

Mean ideal number of sons

Item	Calcutta 1970	Delhi 1968–69	India 1970	Rural East Java 1972	Korea 1971	West Malaysia 1966–67	West Malaysia 1970	Philippines 1968	Taiwan 1967	Belgium 1966	Hungary 1966	United States 1970
Wife's Education												
No formal	2.1	1.9	2.3	2.1	2.5	2.6	2.5	3.5	2.2	—	2.4	*
Primary	1.9	1.8	2.2	1.9	2.2	2.5	2.3	2.8	2.1	1.1	1.1	*
Junior high	1.7	1.7	*	1.6	2.0	2.3	2.0	2.6	1.9	1.2	0.9	1.7
Senior high and over	1.4	1.5	1.9	2.2	1.8	2.0	1.9	2.4	1.8	1.3	0.9	1.4
Urban-Rural Residence												
Large city	*	*	2.0	*	2.0	2.2	2.1	2.5	2.0	1.1	0.8	1.5
Small city	*	*	2.0	*	2.2	2.4	2.3	2.4	2.1	1.2	1.0	1.5
Urban township	*	*	2.1	*	2.1	*	*	2.9	2.2	1.2	1.0	1.5
Rural township	*	*	2.3	*	2.4	2.7	2.4	2.8	2.2	1.3	1.1	1.6
Total	1.8	1.8	2.2	2.0	2.2	2.5	2.4	2.7	2.1	1.2	1.0	1.5
Number of Cases	947	5,242	10,246	411	1,620	4,242	11,918	28,632[a]	4,300	2,566	5,208	4,685

NOTE: See Appendix 1, items 1, 6, and 8 for definitions.
— = Less than 20 cases in the category.
* = No such category.

[a] Frequency weighted as follows: urban respondents × 4 and rural respondents × 12.

be satisfied if desire for a small number of children dominates behavior, the general line of reasoning is that women at a particular stage in family building will have differing attitudes and expectations depending on whether or not they have achieved the sex composition they want. Such differences permit inferences about sex preferences. For example, in Taiwan, among women with three children and no sons, only 8 percent state they want no more children, whereas among those with three children and two or more sons, 69 percent do not want more. Such a relationship does not obtain in the Philippines, another developing country, where about 42 percent of the women with three children want no more children regardless of the number of sons.

The three attitudinal variables for which we have comparative data are: percent who want no more children, number of additional children wanted, and percent who expect more children than they consider ideal. Although these variables are interrelated, they are discussed separately below.

Percent Who Want No More Children

The fact that the percent wanting no more children varies considerably among countries (see Table 1.7) inevitably affects the comparative relationships between the sex distribution of living children and the desire to stop childbearing.[13] In all countries the proportion wanting no more children increases with parity and increases by age within parity and sex composition groups. After age 30, the percent who wish to stop childbearing rises sharply, irrespective of parity. It also increases with age for each sex composition group in most countries, with the exception of those Indian women at higher parities who have no sons. For many countries, however, this detailed comparison is not possible because of the small number of higher parity women with no sons.[14]

In the European countries, beginning with respondents with two living children, the proportion who wish to stop childbearing is quite high

---

[13] Varying definitions and numbers of indeterminates on additional children wanted are discussed in the Introduction and in Appendixes 1 and 2. Most definitions are reasonably similar. But in Ankara, Mexico City, and West Malaysia, 1970, the definition is quite different: women whose present number of children is equal to or greater than their personal ideal are classified as wanting no more children. Although the data for these areas are included in Tables 1.7 and 1.8, they are not really comparable to the other areas.

[14] Although Table 1.8 gives data for the 20–39 year group only, the number of comparisons examined was based on the two age groups, 20–29 and 30–39 years, separately, in order to make a large number of comparisons possible. Comparisons based on the total age group only, however, show a similar clustering of countries.

Table 1.7 Percentage Wanting No More Children and Mean Ideal Number of Children, for Women Aged 20–39 Years

Country, city, or region	Percentage wanting no more children	Mean ideal number of children[a]
West Malaysia, 1966–67	31	4.8
Rural East Java	35	4.2
Jakarta	45	4.9
Mexico City	48	4.0
Philippines	51	*
India	51	3.7
Urban Thailand	51	3.3
Calcutta	54	3.0
Korea	50	3.7
Taiwan	54	3.9
Ankara	56	3.0
Rural Thailand	58	4.0
Great Britain	59	2.7
United States, 1965	64	3.3
Belgium	67	2.6
Hungary	71	2.2

NOTE: See Appendix 1, items 2 and 3 for definitions.
* = No data for this variable.
[a] Means computed from distributions available, with the exception of Calcutta, Taiwan, and the United States. Indeterminates (over 10 percent in India, Malaysia, and Thailand) excluded; assigned values: 0–1 child = 1; 5+ children = 6.

regardless of age of wife (see Table 1.8). With such a high proportion wanting no more children (over 80 percent among older women who have at least two children), there is little room for variation by sex composition. The desire for a small family is the dominating feature. It is at the higher parities that the patterns consistent with our definitions of son preference emerge most strongly. In the developed countries, only a small portion of the population reaches these higher parities.

In such countries as India, Korea, and Taiwan, the presence of one or two sons in the family greatly increases the probability that the woman will consider her family complete and will want no more children. The differences are particularly marked after there are three children in the family. In Korea, for example, 76 percent of third parity women with two or more sons want no more children, as compared with 32 percent of those with one son, and only 15 percent of those with no sons. Unfortunately, we do not know whether those with three children and two or more sons have

Table 1.8 Percentage Wanting No More Children by Number of Living Children and Sons, for Married Women Aged 20–39 Years

Number of living children and sons	Ankara 1966	Calcutta 1970	Delhi 1968–69	India 1970	Rural East Java 1972	Jakarta 1968	Korea 1971	Malaysia 1966–67	Mexico City 1971
None	4	2	14	3	12	15	1	5	3
One child									
No son	5	20	12	20	17	22	8	5	3
One son	0	17	8	14	15	21	5	5	0
Two children	9	22	14	26	18	17	12	5	5
	58	50	49	40	22	28	33	14	13
No son	—	35	19	21	29	26	8	11	—
One son	64	55	58	46	17	24	37	15	19
Two sons	56	49	54	44	22	35	46	12	—
Three children	76	72	71	63	37	47	55	25	36
No son	—	—	27	38	34	—	7	8	—
One son	84	74	67	60	38	43	32	27	31
Two or more sons	69	76	81	68	36	44	76	26	33
Four or more children	80	90	84	86	51	75	81	53	88
No son	—	—	35	40	45	—	13	39	—
One son	76	86	74	76	49	45	54	40	76
Two or more sons	83	91	88	90	52	82	91	56	89
Total	56	54	57	51	35	45	50	31	48
Number of Cases	552	947	5,242	10,246	1,418	811	1,622	4,242	486

NOTE: See Appendix 1, item 3 for definitions.
— = Less than 20 cases in the category.

[a] Frequency is weighted as follows: urban respondents × 4 and rural respondents × 12.

Table 1.8 (Continued)

Number of living children and sons	Philippines 1968	Taiwan 1967	Thailand (urban) 1970	Thailand (rural) 1969	Belgium 1966	Great Britain 1967–68	Hungary 1966	United States 1965
None	0	3	4	14	40	12	27	28
One child	14	4	14	18	59	30	48	31
No son	12	1	15	24	59	29	50	33
One son	16	6	13	12	58	31	46	30
Two children	29	24	38	42	76	76	89	66
No son	24	8	32	27	75	70	84	64
One son	32	26	42	46	77	78	93	70
Two sons	28	31	34	48	76	76	86	61
Three children	41	55	57	58	76	84	92	78
No son	42	8	—	—	80	80	91	81
One son	42	37	54	60	74	86	92	77
Two or more sons	41	69	60	58	77	85	92	79
Four or more children	75	86	80	77	88	86	88	87
No son	68	42	—	—	88	—	—	74
One son	69	65	67	69	92	85	93	87
Two or more sons	77	93	83	80	87	86	88	87
Total	51	54	51	58	67	58	71	64
Number of Cases	28,960[a]	4,300	1,063	642	2,567	1,088	5,309	3,593

any daughters at all. But even if all of them are assumed to have no daughters, we can infer from these data that the drive to have at least one daughter is much weaker than the drive to have at least one son. This is clearly shown by supplementary data from India, especially at the fourth parity. Only 25 percent of women with no daughters want another child, but 79 percent of those with no sons want another. Data from Taiwan show similar results. In none of the four developed countries is the relationship between number of sons and attitude toward further childbearing significant.

Definitions used for sex-preference classifications. To reduce the extensive data from the individual studies to a manageable summary form, a number of conventions have been used that serve a useful function in the absence of more exact measures. The inferences about sex preference from statements about future childbearing are based on the following definitions. If at given parities the percent wanting no more children is higher for those with one or two sons than it is for those with no sons, and if the percent for those with two sons is higher than for those with one, these relationships are defined as being consistent with a preference for sons. Because the open-ended category of two or more sons was used in tabulations, precise information about the number of daughters born to women of third parity and higher is not available. This leads to some ambiguity. For example, it is possible that some of those with two or more sons have no daughters and so want more children in order to have at least one daughter. This does not necessarily mean they have no son preference, but their preference for sons may already be satisfied.

There may also be a preference to have at least one child of each sex. Such a preference for balance can be inferred from these data only in one situation: if, at second parity, the percent wanting no more children is greater for those with one son (and one daughter) than for those with no son or two sons, we define this as indicating a preference for balance. A preference for girls can be inferred if the percent wanting no more children is greater for those with no sons than for those with one or two. Such instances are rarely found in these data.

The inferences from the other variables (such as number of additional children wanted, percent practicing contraception, and percent expecting more children than their ideal) are based on a similar rule about differences. The frequency with which such relationships must occur in order to infer a preference for sons is, of course, a somewhat arbitrary decision. So is the definition of what constitutes a difference as well as the number of cells for which data should be available in order to justify such comparisons. In the following discussion, countries are included in the comparisons if there are sufficient cases to make 50 percent of the appropriate comparisons. Few observed differences are that small, and the relative strength of preference indicated for the various countries would be little changed by a shift in the convention. Nevertheless, caution is required in making comparisons when the differences are small.

Variations among countries. The statistics compared vary on a continuum, and there are no sharp demarcations that would permit us to say that one country is entirely dominated by a son preference and another not. The predominant pattern, however, does vary from one country to another.

The countries that can be compared in regard to the variable "wanting no more children" fall into three clusters. The first includes those for which the relationship indicative of a son preference holds in at least 80 percent of the possible comparisons. These countries, India, Korea, and Taiwan, as well as the city of Delhi, are considered to exhibit a fairly strong preference for sons on this variable (see Table 1.9).

Not all the developing countries show this marked relationship between present family composition and desire for more children. In West Malaysia and urban Thailand, for example, it appears only after the fourth parity and is important only for those with at least two sons. Thus, the second group of developing countries includes those in which the required relationship is found in 50–80 percent of the possible comparisons. West Malaysia, urban Thailand, and Calcutta fall into this group that shows some preference for sons, but not a strong one. Cities within a country may reflect a different system of family values and son preferences from the country as a whole. Pointing up the variations that exist within as well as among countries, for example, Calcutta is quite different from India as a whole, but Delhi is not.

The third cluster includes those countries in which the relationship is found in less than 50 percent of the possible comparisons, primarily the western countries of Great Britain, Belgium, Hungary, and the United States, but also the Philippines and rural East Java.[15] Data for these countries are not consistent with a strong son preference. Java presents a very mixed picture on all variables, partly because of the large indeterminate categories

---

[15] It is by no means certain that the percent of comparisons in which the relationship holds true is the best measure, but it is one way of reducing complex data to a manageable form. The choice of 80 percent and over, 50–80 percent, and less than 50 percent as criteria for grouping countries is arbitrary, but does reflect the clustering that appears on this variable.

Table 1.9 Inferences about Sex Preferences Based on Relationship of Parity and Sex Composition to Percentage Who Want No More Children; Number and Percent of Instances in Which Specified Relationship Holds—Data from Age Groups 20–29 and 30–39

	Son preference[a]		Preference, 1 each sex[a]	
Country, city, or region	Number of comparisons true ÷ number possible	Percent true	Number of comparisons true ÷ number possible	Percent true
Korea	7/7	100	0/2	0
India	12/14	86	1/2	50
Delhi	10/12	83	1/2	50
Taiwan, 1967	10/12	83	1/2	50
West Malaysia, 1966–67	9/14	64	1/2	50
Calcutta	4/7	57	1/1	100
Urban Thailand	4/7	57	1/1	100
Philippines	6/14	43	2/2	100
Great Britain	3/7	43	1/2	50
Rural East Java	4/11	36	1/2	50
Belgium	4/11	36	2/2	100
United States, 1965	4/13	31	1/2	50
Hungary	2/11	18	2/2	100

NOTE: See Appendix 1, item 3 for definitions. Only countries in which at least 7 comparisons (50 percent of total possibilities) can be made are included. Excludes Mexico City, Ankara, Rural Thailand. Comparisons included are counted as exhibiting the relationships specified if differences are as large as 2 percentage points.

[a] Son preference = percent who want no more for those with 1, 2 sons>0 sons; 2 sons>1 son. Preference for 1 of each sex: at parity–2, percent who want no more for 1 son>0, 2 sons. Number of comparisons possible is number of cells with 20+ cases. Total possible for sex preference = 14, for 1 of each sex = 2.

in the study there. But what data there are support the impressionistic view reported by demographers from various parts of Java at a seminar discussion in Jakarta in January 1972 that sex preferences are not strong in Java.

The criterion for a preference for one child of each sex is fully met by second parity women in three developing populations, Calcutta, urban Thailand, and the Philippines, and by Belgium and Hungary among the developed countries. As indicated earlier, however, the test for a preference for a child of each sex can only be applied in these data to second parity women.

Data from the Netherlands are not comparable because they are based on selected marriage cohorts; hence they are not included in the tables with the other comparative material. Further, because of earlier survey indications that sex preference was not important in that culture, questions about preferred sex of children were not asked. (Although there was a supposed desire for one child of each sex, this was considered a "rich man's wish" and not a factor in fertility behavior.) Thus, information on sex of living children was collected in three categories: "boys only," "girls only," and "mixed." The relationship of these categories to the question whether the wife wants more children indicates that the small differences observed (in both the 1958 and 1963 cohorts) are in a direction that corroborates the inference of preference for one child of each sex, an inference somewhat sustained by differential use of contraception and by the parity progression ratios discussed later.

Number of Additional Children Wanted

Further inferences about son preference can be made from the relation of present sex composition to the number of additional children wanted. If son preference is important, women with no sons might be expected to want more additional children than those who already have one or two sons, although the mean number of additional children wanted is relatively small in all countries and differences are necessarily slight, particularly at the higher parities. Such a difference exists in more than 70 percent of the possible comparisons in Korea and Taiwan. In both of these countries third parity women with no sons want an average of 1.1 more children than do those who have two or more sons, a number that is relatively substantial considering the small range possible (see Table 1.10). This contrasts with a difference of 0.1 child or less in the developed countries where present sex composition affects future childbearing desires in less than 18 percent of the possible comparisons.

As with the other variables examined, among the developing countries considerable variation occurs. India as a whole and Delhi and Calcutta assume intermediate positions, although among the older third and fourth parity women the relation of present number of sons to additional children wanted is quite systematic. Although there is certainly not as much evidence of son preference from this variable for India as for Korea and Taiwan, India is much more similar to them than to the developed countries. For other developing countries, such as West Malaysia and Thailand, there is only limited evidence of son preference as related to numbers of additional children wanted. For none of the developed countries is there evidence of son preference on this variable.

Table 1.10 Mean Additional Number of Children Wanted, by Number of Living Children and Sons, for Married Women Aged 20–39 Years

Number of living children and sons	Ankara 1966	Calcutta 1970	Delhi 1968–69	India 1970	Rural East Java 1972	Korea 1971	West Malaysia 1966–67	Mexico City 1971
None	2.7	2.2	2.1	3.0	3.0	2.9	3.4	3.8
One child	1.5	1.1	1.5	2.2	2.7	2.0	3.0	2.4
No son	1.5	1.2	1.5	2.4	2.8	2.2	3.2	2.4
One son	1.5	1.1	1.5	2.1	2.6	1.9	3.0	2.5
Two children	0.7	0.5	0.7	1.4	1.8	1.0	2.6	2.0
No son	—	0.8	1.0	1.4	1.5	1.5	2.9	—
One son	0.6	0.4	0.5	1.6	2.0	0.9	2.5	2.0
Two sons	0.8	0.6	0.5	1.2	1.7	1.0	2.6	—
Three children	0.6	0.1	0.5	1.1	1.6	0.6	2.0	1.2
No son	—	—	0.9	1.3	1.6	1.2	1.7	—
One son	0.4	0.2	0.3	1.2	1.6	0.8	1.9	1.3
Two or more sons	0.7	0.0	0.2	1.0	1.5	0.3	2.0	1.1
Four or more children	0.4	0.1	0.4	0.4	1.9	0.6	1.1	0.4
No son	—	—	0.7	1.0	1.0	1.3	1.9	—
One son	0.5	0.1	0.2	0.5	2.6	0.6	1.5	0.4
Two or more sons	0.4	0.0	0.1	0.4	1.8	0.1	1.0	0.4
Total	0.9	0.6	0.6	1.4	2.2	0.9	2.0	1.3
Number of Cases	552	947	5,242	10,246	1,418	1,622	4,242	486

NOTE: See Appendix 1, item 4 for definitions.   — = Less than 20 cases in the category.

Table 1.10 (Continued)

Number of living children and sons	Taiwan 1967	Thailand (urban) 1970	Thailand (rural) 1969	Belgium 1966	Great Britain 1967–68	Hungary 1966	United States 1965
None	3.1	2.6	2.3	1.2	2.1	1.4	1.8
One child	2.2	1.5	2.0	0.6	1.0	0.6	1.1
No son	2.4	1.4	2.3	0.6	1.0	0.5	1.1
One son	2.1	1.6	1.8	0.6	1.0	0.6	1.2
Two children	1.2	1.0	1.3	0.3	0.3	0.1	0.5
No son	1.8	1.0	1.3	0.4	0.4	0.2	0.5
One son	1.1	0.9	1.6	0.3	0.3	0.1	0.4
Two sons	1.0	1.0	0.9	0.3	0.3	0.1	0.6
Three children	0.6	0.6	0.6	0.3	0.1	0.1	0.3
No son	1.6	—	—	0.3	0.2	0.1	0.2
One son	0.7	0.6	0.6	0.3	0.1	0.1	0.3
Two or more sons	0.4	0.5	—	0.2	0.1	0.1	0.3
Four or more children	0.2	0.2	0.3	0.1	0.1	0.1	0.2
No son	0.9	—	—	0.0	—	—	0.5
One son	0.4	0.3	0.4	0.1	0.2	0.1	0.2
Two or more sons	0.1	0.1	0.4	0.1	0.1	0.1	0.2
Total	0.8	0.8	0.9	0.5	0.7	0.3	0.6
Number of Cases	4,300	1,063	642	2,567	1,088	5,309	3,593

From these data, of course, we do not know whether the additional children desired are boys or girls. Supplementary data from India and Taiwan show that women with no sons report a higher mean number of sons wanted than those with no daughters report daughters wanted. This is true until fifth parity is reached. Regardless of the number or sex composition of present living children, in almost every instance a greater number of additional sons than daughters is wanted. Except among those with no sons, however, differences are rather small. Again, the data indicate that daughters are wanted as well as sons, but not to the same extent.

Percent Who Expect More Children Than They Consider Ideal

Some women may expect to have more children than they personally consider ideal, either because of ineffective fertility control or for other reasons. If a high value is placed on sons, some women may expect to go beyond their ideal number if they have not had the desired sons. The level of this phenomenon varies considerably by country, from a low of 6 percent in rural East Java to a high of 58 percent in Mexico City. With respect to this variable, comparisons are possible for only six of the populations, and even for these, some definitional differences remain.[16]

All the countries for which we have data, however, fall into a pattern similar to that based on previous indicators: a son preference inference is supported for Korea and Taiwan; it is not supported in the United States, Belgium, Hungary, and rural East Java, with urban Thailand falling in between. Calcutta, which was classified previously as more intermediate in son preference, appears more consistent with a fairly strong son preference on the basis of expecting more children than considered ideal. The strength of son preference in Taiwan and Korea is demonstrated by the relatively high proportion of third and fourth parity women with no sons who expect to have more children than they consider ideal. In Taiwan, 25 percent of third parity and 48 percent of fourth parity women with no sons expect to exceed their ideal family size. In Korea, the corresponding figures are 68 and 95 percent. The proportions are much smaller for those who have two or more sons (see Table 1.11).

An inference of a preference for one child of each sex among second parity women is not supported on this variable for any of the countries except Hungary and urban Thailand, and there only for the younger women.

---

[16] Being compound, this variable is related to both the level of expected family size and the personal ideal for family size, and for both of these components definitions vary in these data. See Appendix 1 for details of definitions used. Data on this variable were unavailable for Delhi, West Malaysia, the Philippines, and Great Britain.

Table 1.11 Percentage Who Expect More Than Ideal, by Number of Living Children and Sons, for Married Women Aged 20–39 Years

Number of living children and sons	Ankara 1966	Calcutta 1970	Rural East Java 1972	Korea 1971	Mexico City 1971	Taiwan 1967	Thailand (urban) 1970	Thailand (rural) 1969	Belgium 1966	Hungary 1966	United States 1965
None	19	2	1	7	12	0	2	0	1	3	4
One child	32	2	2	15	28	1	5	8	5	3	8
No son	31	4	1	19	33	1	8	9	5	2	10
One son	33	1	3	12	25	0	3	8	5	4	7
Two children	39	2	5	14	42	4	8	12	11	8	12
No son	—	5	4	29	—	4	16	4	8	7	10
One son	40	1	5	10	38	5	5	20	10	6	12
Two sons	35	2	6	8	—	3	8	4	16	11	14
Three children	60	10	6	23	48	11	18	9	35	39	24
No son	—	—	3	68	—	25	—	—	30	48	29
One son	62	13	8	35	45	14	18	8	35	34	27
Two or more sons	56	9	5	10	48	8	15	9	36	40	21
Four or more children	77	68	9	57	84	9	39	40	55	67	50
No son	—	—	0	95	—	48	—	—	50	—	51
One son	82	67	5	72	71	25	46	29	45	68	44
Two or more sons	77	68	10	51	86	4	38	42	58	65	52
Total	52	23	6	32	58	7	21	24	17	12	22
Number of Cases	552	947	1,418	1,622	486	4,300	1,063	642	2,567	5,309	3,593

NOTE: See Appendix 1, item 5 for definitions.   — = Less than 20 cases in the category.

Behavioral Evidence

In the populations considered in this study, data are available on two behavioral variables that are indicators of sex preference: percent currently practicing contraception and parity progression ratios.

Percent Currently Practicing Contraception

If sex preference exists, then the practice of contraception should be related to the size and sex composition of the family. If the desired number of sons or daughters have already been born, presumably women will be more inclined to practice contraception, particularly if they do so for limiting, rather than spacing, births.

Level of contraceptive use varies widely by country, from less than 10 percent in West Malaysia and Jakarta (for all women aged 20–39 years) to more than 70 percent in all western countries represented here (see Table 1.12). Among the developing countries, only in Korea and Taiwan are as many as 25 percent of the women practicing contraception. Where the level of practice is very low, for example below 15 percent as in India, West Malaysia, rural Thailand, and the Philippines, there is less room for variation with differing sex composition.

The possible effect of the *level* of contraceptive use in the population on the relation between the number and sex distribution of children and contraceptive practice is well illustrated in the contrast between India as a whole and the city of Delhi. In India, which exhibits strong son preference in attitudinal statements, the presence of sons is not consistently related to use of contraception; in only 57 percent of the possible comparisons is the use of contraception greater among those with more sons (see Table 1.13). The level of contraceptive use is low, never rising above 20 percent, except among those with five or more children. In Delhi, however, where the overall level of use is as high as 47 percent, the relationship of the son preference exhibited in other variables is clearly reflected also in the proportion using contraception. In 92 percent of the possible comparisons, those with more sons were more apt to be practicing contraception. Perhaps contraceptive use must be above some threshold level before expressed preferences are reflected in behavior. If the practice of contraception is begun late, for example after four or five births, then the possibility of a relation to sex distribution at lower parities is very small, and by the higher parities, most women will have their desired sex distributions.

Calcutta, Thailand, and Malaysia are in the middle range on this variable, a position consistent with their expressed preferences. In Belgium, Great Britain, Hungary, and the United States, there is the least evidence for a son preference as measured by practice of contraception, again a behavioral position that is consistent with expressed preferences and attitudes toward having additional children.

In the developed countries, where contraception is widely practiced for spacing births, the practice of contraception is a poorer indicator of sex preference than in developing countries, where contraception usually is begun only after all the children wanted are born. In both groups of countries, insofar as contraception is practiced, it is reasonable to suppose that women who are satisfied with the number and sex composition of their children would be most likely to use contraception. However, especially in the developed countries, women not so satisfied might also use contraception to space their children in the expectation that a desired son or daughter could be born later. The question of the purpose of contraceptive use is thus a complicating factor in comparing behavior in countries where contraception is used almost entirely for limiting births with those in which there is widespread use for spacing.

Parity Progression Ratios

If the wish to have sons is very strong in a culture, we might expect that among couples with a specified number of children there would be a relationship between the sex distribution of those children and the contingent probability of going on to the next parity. Those who do not yet have the desired sons would be more apt to proceed to the next parity. This behavioral pattern, of course, presupposes that a sufficient number of women do something to control their fertility in accordance with their preferences.

Data on parity progressions are available for Korea, Taiwan, India, West Malaysia, rural East Java, Hungary, Great Britain, and the United States, countries already discussed with regard to the other variables. In addition, data are available for Mexico City and Ankara, cities for which the survey data on the previous variables produced too few cases in many cells to be useful for comparative purposes.

The criteria used for inferring a son preference from parity progression ratios are as follows: (1) among women who have reached a given parity, those who have all daughters are more apt to go on to the next parity than those with all sons, and (2) those with more daughters than sons are more apt to go on to the next parity than those with more sons than daughters.

Table 1.12 Percentage Currently Using Contraception, by Number of Living Children and Sons, for Married Women Aged 20–39 Years

Number of living children and sons	Ankara[a] 1966	Calcutta 1970	Delhi 1968–69	India 1970	Rural East Java 1972	Jakarta 1968	Korea 1971	West Malaysia 1966–67	Mexico City 1971
None	11	16	4	2	1	1	0	3	13
One child	36	43	29	6	4	6	5	7	23
No son	31	37	27	6	1	7	1	7	25
One son	39	47	30	6	6	3	8	7	22
Two children	48	44	52	12	4	6	15	6	27
No son	—	37	47	8	2	9	5	8	—
One son	50	47	53	10	5	6	16	6	31
Two sons	44	45	54	17	3	5	21	4	—
Three children	44	46	58	13	14	11	29	12	28
No son	—	—	42	18	12	—	15	8	—
One son	42	60	55	10	16	14	19	10	26
Two or more sons	44	41	62	15	14	10	36	13	29
Four or more children	29	42	59	19	17	14	36	12	22
No son	—	—	54	13	18	—	13	3	—
One son	29	35	61	20	15	16	26	7	38
Two or more sons	27	44	59	19	17	15	40	13	20
Total	37	40	47	12	11	9	24	9	24
Number of cases	552	947	5,242	10,246	1,418	811	1,622	4,242	486

NOTE: Sterilization included as contraception except in Belgium and Great Britain.
— = Less than 20 cases in the category.

[a] Defined as "ever used contraception."
[b] Frequency is weighted as follows: urban respondents × 4 and rural respondents × 12.

Table 1.12 (Continued)

Number of living children and sons	Philippines 1968	Taiwan 1967	Thailand (urban) 1970	Thailand (rural) 1969	Belgium 1966	Great Britain 1967-68	Hungary 1966	United States 1965
None	0	4	11	0	49	55	30	42
One child								
No son	12	4	28	7	75	62	70	56
One son	15	2	24	3	76	63	71	52
One son	9	5	31	10	75	62	68	58
Two children								
No son	14	20	39	8	82	82	80	79
One son	14	6	34	4	81	86	81	80
One son	16	21	43	8	84	80	80	78
Two sons	11	26	32	11	81	84	79	80
Three children								
No son	20	36	54	17	81	86	76	81
No son	19	8	—	—	82	82	77	85
One son	19	27	52	18	78	86	77	79
Two or more sons	20	43	54	14	83	87	76	82
Four or more children								
No son	17	47	53	17	82	68	58	80
No son	23	24	—	—	69	—	—	91
One son	18	39	47	14	87	82	68	78
Two or more sons	17	49	55	18	82	64	56	80
Total	15	32	43	13	76	72	74	72
Number of cases	28,960[b]	4,300	1,063	642	2,567	1,088	5,309	3,593

Table 1.13 Summary of Evidence for Sex Preference Based on Relationship of Parity and Sex Composition to Five Variables

Country, city, or region	Son preference[a]					Preference, 1 each sex[a]				
	V1	V2	V3	V4	V5	V1	V2	V3	V4	V5
Korea	100	100	100	60	71	0	0	0	0	100
India	86	*	57	42	57	50	*	0	25	0
Delhi	83	*	92	54	54	50	*	0	0	0
Taiwan, 1967	83	75	71	85	83	50	0	50	0	0
Ankara	*	*	*	78	*	*	*	*	25	*
Mexico City	*	*	*	70	*	*	*	*	25	*
West Malaysia, 1966–67	64	*	43	67	50	50	*	*	25	0
Calcutta	57	71	43	*	43	100	0	100	*	100
Urban Thailand	57	57	50	*	43	100	100	0	*	100
Philippines	43	*	21	*	*	100	*	50	*	*
Great Britain	43	*	57	17	14	50	*	0	100	0
Rural East Java	36	18	45	54	45	50	0	50	33	0
Belgium	36	9	27	*	18	100	0	50	*	0
United States, 1965	31	31	38	40	0	50	0	0	33	50
Hungary	18	9	27	20	0	100	50	50	0	0

NOTE: V1 = Percent wanting no more children.
V2 = Percent expecting more than their ideal.
V3 = Percent currently using contraception.
V4 = Parity progression ratios.
V5 = Number of additional children wanted.
* = No data for this variable, or insufficient data cells for comparisons.
[a] Relevant comparisons are similar to those cited in Table 1.9.

Other criteria might be possible—that at fourth parity those with more daughters than sons would be more apt to go on than those with equal sons and daughters, and than those with all sons. This latter comparison is possible in only six of the ten countries being compared. If the former criterion is added, it would reduce somewhat the relative strength of the inference indicated below about son preference in Mexico City.

The criterion used for evidence of a preference for one child of each sex is: if, among women who have reached second parity, those who have equal numbers of sons and daughters are less apt to go on to the next parity than others, then such a preference is indicated.

Comparisons of the parity progression ratios shown in Table 1.14 support the inference of a son preference in Korea, Taiwan, West Malaysia,

Mexico City, and Ankara, but not in India, rural East Java, Great Britain, Hungary, or the United States. In the former group, the evidence in 60 percent or more of the possible comparisons supports son preference. In Great Britain, the evidence in only 17 percent does. Only the data from Great Britain support the inference of a preference for one child of each sex, and even there the differences are small.

That interpretations made on the basis of the parity progression ratio differences may vary, depending on auxiliary data, was suggested by the Indian investigators. For example, a fourth parity woman with no sons may stop childbearing, not because she has no preference for sons but because the fear of having another daughter may outweigh the hope for a son. This may be particularly pertinent in a culture where dowries for daughters are important.

As discussed earlier, the parities at which sex preferences affect further childbearing may vary with the culture. Where almost everyone goes on to have more than two children, the sex composition of the two-child family may be of less importance as a determinant of continued childbearing. Nevertheless, in most developing countries, even the comparisons among those with two children (Table 1.14) are consistent with the inferences of a son preference made from data on attitudes and behavior presented earlier.

In countries with moderately high ideal family size, the pertinent parity is probably the third or fourth. If only third parity is considered, the pattern is always in favor of a son preference in Korea, Malaysia, and Taiwan, and among older women in India. The situation in Mexico City and Ankara points up another issue. Unless sample sizes are large, the probability is that by third and fourth parity the number of cases with no sons or no daughters will be very small, and comparisons cannot be made. For these two cities, the data for those with only sons or daughters have been combined with data for the adjacent categories (for example, all female combined with more female than male). Consequently, fewer comparisons are possible.

In drawing conclusions from parity progression ratios, three other factors should be borne in mind. The first has already been mentioned: a reasonable level of contraceptive use must exist before conclusions about son preference can be made on the basis of the probability of going on to the next parity. In this regard, the chronology of family planning practice may be important. In retrospective data such as these, many of the women in the developing countries were at the early parities prior to any widespread use of family planning. The fact that they did not then have the means to control their fertility in accordance with possible preferences does not mean that such preferences did not exist at that time. As practice of

Table 1.14 Parity Progression Ratios, by Wife's Age and Sex of Living Children, for Married Women Aged 20-39 Years Who Have Reached Specified Parities

Wife's age (years) and sex of living children	Ankara[b] 1966			Rural East Java 1972			India 1970			Korea 1971			West Malaysia 1966-67		
	2	3	4	2	3	4	2	3	4	2	3	4	2	3	4
20-29															
All female	68	61	46	66	47	34	51	41	35	48	14	10	57	49	52
Female>male	77	—	—	69	45	—	47	39	22	52	32	—	61	56	77
Female=male	66	65	46	65	43	50	—	41	36	—	12	—	—	51	52
Male>female	—	57	50	—	56	25	58	—	23	47	—	—	56	—	50
All male	63	—	41	67	37	32	—	41	45	42	11	—	—	44	42
				—	—	—	46	47	70	—	0	—	54	52	53
30-39															
All female	82	71	66	90	32	71	81	74	60	87	72	53	87	82	71
Female>male	98	74	70	88	36	67	83	80	78	89	84	57	90	86	79
Female=male	—	—	—	—	32	70	—	76	63	—	73	72	—	84	69
Male>female	76	68	66	93	32	66	78	71	57	86	72	55	86	79	67
All male	81	—	62	86	30	78	83	71	60	87	60	36	85	78	71
				—	—	79	—	—	57	—	—	—	—	—	84
20-39															
All female	76	67	58	80	59	62	65	60	53	74	60	51	75	72	67
Female>male	88	70	61	80	71	60	63	65	67	73	69	44	79	78	79
Female=male	—	—	—	—	58	66	—	60	56	—	59	66	—	74	66
Male>female	71	63	60	80	72	54	66	58	47	74	63	55	74	70	64
All male	74	—	54	77	55	66	66	64	55	74	44	36	73	71	66
				—	—	76	—	—	59	—	—	—	—	—	76

— = Less than 20 cases in the category.

[a] For space reasons, parities 1 and 5 or more are omitted.

[b] Data based on number of children ever born. Because of insufficient cases, parities 3 and 4 "all female" and "female>male" are combined, as are "all male" and "male>female."

[c] Data based on number of children ever born. Data do not extend to parity 4.

Table 1.14 (Continued)

Wife's age (years) and sex of living children	Mexico City[b] 1971			Taiwan 1967			Great Britain[c] 1967–68		Hungary 1966			United States 1965		
	2	3	4	2	3	4	2	3	2	3	4	2	3	4
20–29														
All female	72	62	60	56	37	21	30	31	24	32	30	53	42	34
Female>male	65			60	47	40	30	—	32	30	20	57	52	—
Female=male		61	63		40	26		—		31	10		37	35
Male>female	75	63	64	54	33	16	27	41	22	31	37	50	45	36
All male	70		53	56	34	30	35	—	19	36	56	55	38	27
30–39														
All female	86	88	87	93	80	58	50	43	39	38	47	70	58	54
Female>male	95			96	93	80	51	36	41	30	80	70	51	53
Female=male		89	86		86	69		46		34	41		58	54
Male>female	80		92	93	73	53	47	42	38	39	46	70	59	55
All male	92	86	82	92	72	48	53	38	40	48	67	71	63	60
20–39														
All female	80	77	78	78	67	52	43	40	35	36	44	63	53	49
Female>male	80			82	80	75	44	27	38	30	65	65	52	48
Female=male		78	79		72	62		43		34	34		51	48
Male>female	78	76	82	77	61	47	40	42	34	38	44	62	55	50
All male	83		72	78	61	45	46	35	34	46	59	65	55	58

contraception increases, we would expect the influence of a son preference, where it exists, to be felt increasingly.

Another pertinent factor is that in countries where child mortality is, or recently has been, high, women may go on to have another child to replace a specific child who died, rather than because they wanted to satisfy a sex preference. This could obscure the relationship under study. In the Taiwan data presented, in order to minimize this problem, the analysis was confined to those women who had not experienced a child death prior to the particular parity under consideration. This more complicated computer procedure was not carried out with the other data sets. Taiwan data were computed by both procedures. Although of potential importance, the results as far as inferences of sex preferences are concerned differed little for the two methods.

Marriage duration also affects the probability that a couple will have had a specified number of children. Since this factor is not controlled in these data, we may assume that some, particularly among the younger women, may not have moved to the next parity because they have not been married a sufficient time, rather than because of any considerations of family sex composition. Here the data from the Netherlands, based on marriage cohorts, are particularly pertinent. Even though all women have had equal time to reach selected parities, no evidence of selective behavior based on preference for a given sex of child emerged, either for the 1958 or 1963 cohorts. In an examination of the Taiwan data, controlling for marriage duration did not change the relationship of numbers of sons to parity progression ratios, but in other countries the relationships might be altered if marriage duration were taken into consideration.

Conclusion

In reviewing the evidence for sex preference provided by the comparative data brought together in this project, the measurement problems stemming from the kinds of variables available in the usual fertility studies become apparent. Because adequate direct measures of sex preference are not available, indirect measures and inferences from attitudinal and behavioral statements must be used. Not only are these cumbersome for cross-population comparisons, but there is often an overlap and possible confusion in using behavioral variables to index both preferences and the behavior that may be related to preferences. Nevertheless, the available data permit a number of interesting and valuable comparisons. The countries have been placed for summary purposes in three broad groups with respect to the preference for sons, but our discussion should have made it clear that some of the countries could be moved from one group to another, depending on the criteria emphasized.

One salient point, however, is clear. While there are great differences between the developed and developing countries on this issue, there are also major differences among the developing countries for which we have data. A consistent or marked preference for sons was not found in any of the developed countries, and it was found only in some of the developing countries.

Most of the evidence from stated preferences and attitudes indicates that in Korea and Taiwan, and to a slightly lesser extent in India and Delhi, there is a reasonably clear preference for sons. Nevertheless, it should be kept in mind that in no country do the data indicate a desire for sons to the exclusion of daughters. In none of these countries is there evidence for a preference by any significant number for just one child of each sex. Behavior, however, does not always mesh with attitudes. In Korea and Taiwan, the practice of contraception and the parity progression ratios are consistent with a preference for sons; so too are the parity progression ratios in Mexico City and Ankara, the only variable for which we have sufficient comparative data for those areas. In Delhi, the relatively high use of contraception among women with more sons is consistent with their expressed preferences and attitudes toward having additional children. For India as a whole this is not the case, however, particularly among the younger women.

A second group of populations can be delineated—developing countries in which there appears to be some preference for sons on some criteria but not on others. Calcutta, West Malaysia, the Philippines, and Thailand occupy this middle position. In this group, stated preferences are available only for West Malaysia. There, the preferred number of children and the preferred number of sons are quite high, and the proportions wanting no more children and those using contraception are the lowest of any of the countries examined. Under these conditions, any preference for sons that exists appears to have little impact on behavior. It might appear at high parities if the desired sex composition had not been achieved, but the probabilities are that at the later stages of family building the desired number of sons would have been born.

In the third group, the western countries represented here by Belgium, Great Britain, Hungary, and the United States, there is no systematic indication of sex preference, either in attitudinal statements or in behavior.

TWO

Practice of Contraception by Women Wanting No More Children

During the demographic transition from high to low fertility that usually follows mortality decline, presumably there must be a period during which many couples of childbearing age have come to want no more children but have not yet adopted effective birth control practices. Unless we assume that the gradual development of a new value—wanting fewer births—is immediately followed by the adoption of birth control, we can expect a group to exist with discrepant goals and means. This should be a group with a high potential for adopting contraception or other means of birth control and for reducing fertility.

Therefore, the size and correlates of the discrepant group are of considerable importance. One way to identify these couples from survey data is to single out those who say they want no more children but are not practicing contraception. The size of the group will depend on two components: (1) the proportion who want no more children, and among them (2) the proportion who are not practicing contraception. The Population Council has previously collected comparative data on the two components,[1] but the components have not been considered jointly and comparatively to assess the size and correlates of the discrepant group that may indicate a potential for change in fertility and family planning. That was the objective of this part of the IUSSP comparative project.

---

[1] D. Nortman, "Population and family planning programs: A factbook," *Reports on Population/Family Planning*, no. 2 (5th ed.), (September 1973).

We find in surveys in the developing countries that many couples say they want no more children but still are not practicing contraception. The significance of this fact as an indicator of potential contraceptive use depends partly on the degree of confidence in the survey responses about additional children wanted, an issue that will be taken up later in the discussion of the findings of this comparative analysis.

In this analysis we will concentrate on women over age 30 years. By that age a large proportion (usually a majority) of women in all populations say that they want no more children, so the salience of contraception should be greatest then. Further, it was use of birth control by women over age 30 that first reduced the birth rates in most of the countries that have reached low fertility levels.[2] In addition, concentration on women over age 30 reduces the effects of widely differing ages of marriage among the countries compared. The variation in the proportion of an age cohort not represented in the samples because they are still unmarried is a less serious problem at the older ages.

Overview

Among women over age 30 in the countries in this study, the proportion who want no more children but are not practicing contraception is much greater in developing than in developed countries, but the range of variation among developing countries is considerable (Table 2.1). The major source of these differences is not in the proportion who want no more; it is in the proportion who are practicing contraception among those who want no more (compare rows 1 and 3 in Table 2.1). As we will see, in some developing countries with a high desired number of children the proportion who want no more children is relatively low until many children are born. But, overall, the major differences are in the practice of contraception among those who say they want no more children.

Table 2.2 illustrates some of the different combinations of the two components that produce the variations observed. In Taiwan[3] and West Malaysia the nearly identical proportions in the discrepant group result

---

[2] United Nations, *The Determinants and Consequences of Population Trends* (New York: United Nations, 1973), Chapter IV.

[3] By 1970 the proportion who wanted no more children and were not using contraception had declined considerably in Taiwan. Although data for Taiwan, 1970, are included in a number of tables to illustrate trends, the discussion refers to the 1967 data unless otherwise indicated.

Table 2.1 Ranges in Percents Wanting No More Children, Practicing Contraception, Not Practicing Contraception Among Those Who Want No More Children, and Not Practicing Contraception and Wanting No More Children, for Developed and Developing Countries, for Women Aged 30–39 Years

Item	Developing countries	Developed countries
Percent who want no more children	43–78[a]	79–82
Percent practicing contraception	11–48	70–85
Percent not practicing contraception among those who want no more children	27–89	8–21
Percent not practicing contraception *and* want no more children	21–54	6–19

NOTE: See Appendix 1, item 3 for definitions. Sterilization included as contraception except in Belgium and Great Britain.

[a] Range is 62–78 if West Malaysia is excluded.

Table 2.2 Comparison of Selected Developed and Developing Countries with Respect to Percent Wanting No More Children, Practicing Contraception, Not Practicing Contraception Among Those Who Want No More Children, and Not Practicing Contraception and Wanting No More Children, for Women Aged 30–39 Years

	Countries			
Item	India 1970	Taiwan 1967	Malaysia 1966–67	Belgium 1966
Percent who want no more children	67	78	43	79
Percent practicing contraception	15	55	11	76
Percent not practicing contraception among those who want no more children	80	45	80	12
Percent not practicing contraception *and* want no more children	54	35	34	10

NOTE: See Appendix 1, item 3 for definitions. Sterilization included as contraception except in Belgium and Great Britain.

from very different combinations of the two components. Taiwan has a much higher percentage who want no more children, but, since it also has a much higher percentage practicing contraception, the net results are almost identical with those in West Malaysia with respect to percentage who want no more and are not practicing contraception. Belgium has a very low percentage who want no more children and are not practicing contraception, because, while the large majority want no more, among them a very large proportion are practicing contraception. Compare India and Taiwan. Although the percentage who want no more children is somewhat larger in Taiwan than in India, the percentage among the Taiwanese women practicing contraception is so much greater that Taiwan has substantially fewer of the "discrepant" cases—that is, those who want no more children and are not practicing contraception.

Although mainly a phenomenon among women over 30, the size of the discrepant group among women of all ages (20–39) is greater in all of the developing populations than in any of the developed populations. For the developing populations the range is from 16 percent (Delhi) to 50 percent (rural Thailand) (see Table 2.6, p. 56). This compares with the lower values and smaller range of 5 to 14 percent (Great Britain and Hungary) in the developed countries.

The data available for the populations considered in this study permit analysis of practice of contraception by women wanting no more children in terms of three variables: age of wife, parity, and wife's education. We will consider each in turn and then discuss the validity and reliability of the data.

Variations with Wife's Age

In all countries, developed and developing, the percentage who want no more children increases fairly rapidly with wife's age (Table 2.3). By age 30–34 in all countries except West Malaysia a majority of respondents, ranging from 55 to 77 percent, say they want no more children. By age 35–39 the percentages rise further to a range of 67 to 90 percent (again excepting West Malaysia). At ages 25–29 the percentage who want no more children is higher in the developed countries (46–55 percent) than in any of the developing countries (21–45 percent, excluding the developing cities), but the differences among some of the countries in the two groups are only 1 or 2 percent. At ages 20–24 and 30–39 the ranges for the two groups of populations overlap.

The difference between the developed and developing countries is much greater with respect to the practice of contraception at all age levels, whether among all women or among those who want no more children (Tables 2.4 and 2.5). At age 20–24 in the developing populations, from

Table 2.3 Percentage Wanting No More Children, by Wife's Age and Number of Living Children, for Married Women Aged 20–39 Years

Wife's age (years) and number of living children	Ankara 1966	Calcutta 1970	India 1970	Korea 1971	West Malaysia 1966–67	West Malaysia 1970	Mexico City 1971	Philippines 1968
20–24	36	23	24	7	12	9	18	20
25–29	59	44	44	25	21	24	46	42
30–34	57	65	62	60	34	36	57	57
35–39	67	80	73	85	54	36	69	72
Total	56	54	51	50	31	26	48	51
20–29								
<2 children	50	36	35	19	17	17	34	34
2	6	8	9	4	3	1	4	8
3	58	34	36	23	12	11	2	25
4	71	60	57	43	22	17	15	40
5 or more	84	82	82	38	42	46	36	59
	—	—	80	—	50	56	88	77
30–39								
<2 children	62	72	67	72	43	36	63	64
2	2	24	23	18	13	3	—	13
3	59	74	48	53	17	20	11	38
4	80	83	69	64	28	24	35	43
5 or more	69	92	84	77	40	53	88	62
	85	91	90	88	60	46		83
20–39								
<2 children	56	54	51	50	31	26	48	51
2	5	17	13	6	5	1	3	9
3	58	50	40	33	14	14	3	29
4	76	72	63	55	25	20	14	41
5 or more	74	88	83	74	41	50	36	61
	88	91	88	87	58	48	88	82
Number of Cases	552	947	10,246	1,622	4,242	13,449	486	28,964[b]

NOTE: See Appendix 1, item 3 for definitions.
— = Less than 20 cases in the category.
[a] Taiwan 1970 data refer to ages 22–39.
[b] Frequency is weighted as follows: urban respondents × 4 and rural respondents × 12.

Table 2.3 (Continued)

Wife's age (years) and number of living children	Taiwan 1967	Taiwan[a] 1970	Thailand (urban) 1970	Thailand (rural) 1969	Belgium 1966	Great Britain 1967–68	Hungary 1966	United States 1965
20–24	10	13	23	32	30	19	29	33
25–29	35	38	38	45	46	46	55	55
30–34	70	77	56	60	69	75	77	74
35–39	87	92	70	74	86	88	90	88
Total	54	61	50	58	67	58	66	64
20–29	26	32	32	40	42	34	51	44
<2 children	6	0	10	16	25	7	31	14
2	19	19	32	41	66	60	84	53
3	44	53	53	54	68	79	86	66
4	70	66	77	62	81	—	86	77
5 or more	87	83	91	—	—	—	—	85
30–39	78	84	62	68	79	82	85	81
<2 children	22	37	12	18	74	62	71	60
2	43	56	47	46	80	88	92	80
3	66	80	59	62	77	87	93	87
4	84	88	76	68	93	88	92	90
5 or more	92	94	82	84	85	86	86	89
20–39	54	61	50	58	67	58	71	64
<2 children	34	5	11	16	53	23	48	30
2	24	28	38	42	76	76	89	66
3	55	64	57	58	76	84	92	78
4	81	82	76	66	91	85	90	85
5 or more	91	93	83	83	85	87	85	88
Number of Cases	4,300	2,491	1,080	642	2,567	1,088	5,309	3,593

Table 2.4 Percentage Currently Using Contraception, by Wife's Age and Number of Living Children, for Married Women Aged 20–39 Years

Wife's age (years) and number of living children	Ankara[a] 1966	Calcutta 1970	India 1970	Korea 1971	West Malaysia 1966-67	West Malaysia 1970	Mexico City 1971	Philippines 1968
20-24	25	31	7	2	5	14	19	10
25-29	37	42	12	15	9	20	26	16
30-34	43	44	13	28	10	20	24	18
35-39	40	43	16	37	12	18	25	16
Total	37	40	12	24	9	18	24	15
20-29								
<2 children	42	38	10	10	7	17	23	14
2	28	37	5	4	5	10	16	8
3	40	39	10	12	5	19	24	13
4	39	36	13	22	10	21	23	17
5 or more	19	40	12	15	10	21	23	18
	—	—	30	—	10	22	25	14
30-39								
<2 children	41	43	15	33	11	19	25	17
2	23	25	4	2	5	8	—	5
3	59	52	13	20	8	16	36	16
4	49	57	14	34	12	18	36	22
5 or more	45	44	15	40	10	18	21	17
	21	42	22	34	13	22		17
20-39								
<2 children	37	40	12	24	9	18	24	15
2	26	33	5	3	5	10	13	7
3	48	44	12	15	6	18	23	14
4	44	46	13	29	12	20	27	20
5 or more	36	42	14	38	10	18	28	18
	18	42	24	35	13	22	22	16
Number of Cases	552	947	10,246	1,622	4,242	13,449	486	28,964[c]

NOTE: Sterilization included as contraception except in Belgium and Great Britain.
— = Less than 20 cases in the category.
[a] Defined as "ever used contraception."
[b] Taiwan 1970 data refer to ages 22–39.
[c] Frequency is weighted as follows: urban respondents × 4 and rural respondents × 12.

Table 2.4 (Continued)

Wife's age (years) and number of living children	Taiwan 1967	Taiwan[b] 1970	Thailand (urban) 1970	Thailand (rural) 1969	Belgium 1966	Great Britain 1967–68	Hungary 1966	United States 1965
20–24	6	13	24	6	68	65	64	62
25–29	23	30	40	11	76	72	70	70
30–34	41	55	51	17	78	74	72	76
35–39	50	63	44	14	75	75	69	77
Total	32	44	42	13	76	72	69	72
20–29	16	26	36	9	74	69	74	66
<2 children	3	6	22	3	68	59	71	51
2	15	26	35	9	83	81	81	76
3	26	32	46	15	89	84	70	74
4	34	44	52	18	67	—	49	82
5 or more	43	41	70	—	—	—	—	75
30–39	45	58	48	16	76	75	85	76
<2 children	7	18	22	8	67	60	66	49
2	36	39	43	6	82	83	80	83
3	46	61	58	19	79	86	78	86
4	52	62	50	16	87	72	64	84
5 or more	46	62	53	18	80	64	54	78
20–39	32	44	42	13	76	72	74	72
<2 children	4	8	22	4	68	59	69	50
2	20	28	39	8	82	82	80	79
3	36	46	54	17	81	86	76	81
4	48	58	50	16	84	71	61	84
5 or more	46	60	54	17	79	64	54	77
Number of Cases	4,300	2,491	1,080	642	2,567	1,088	5,309	3,593

Table 2.5 Of Those Who Want No More Children, Percentage Not Using Contraception, by Wife's Age and Number of Living Children, for Married Women Aged 20–39 Years

Wife's age (years) and number of living children	Ankara[a] 1966	Calcutta 1970	Delhi[b] 1968–69	India 1970	Rural East Java 1972	Jakarta 1968	Korea 1971	West Malaysia 1966–67	Mexico City 1971
20–24	73	58	43	85	43	90	—	95	68
25–29	61	45	30	78	65	89	70	84	67
30–34	49	46	26	81	65	87	59	80	78
35–39	55	52	28	79	81	90	56	81	72
Total	58	49	29	80	69	89	60	82	72
20–29	64	48	33	80	61	89	73	87	68
<2 children	—	—	58	86	54	93	100	100	—
2	55	41	26	79	76	92	81	86	—
3	55	52	30	81	52	81	66	82	—
4	85	51	34	86	60	93	60	84	—
5 or more	—	—	45	68	70	81	—	86	72
30–39	53	49	27	80	73	89	58	80	75
<2 children	—	62	72	93	100	98	—	96	—
2	39	41	24	78	91	96	68	83	—
3	46	41	20	80	71	80	54	74	—
4	48	51	22	83	72	63	50	83	—
5 or more	78	55	27	75	67	82	62	80	78
20–39	58	49	29	80	69	89	60	82	72
<2 children	—	43	67	89	82	95	96	98	—
2	48	41	25	79	83	93	74	90	—
3	50	46	24	81	61	81	58	78	—
4	62	51	26	84	68	76	50	83	65
5 or more	82	55	29	74	67	82	61	81	76
Number of Cases[c]	310	511	3,009	5,195	491	367	797	1,302	234

NOTE: See Appendix 1, item 3 for definitions. Sterilization included as contraception except in Belgium and Great Britain.
— = Less than 20 cases in the category.

[a] Defined as "of those wanting no more children, percent never used contraception."
[b] Taiwan 1970 data refer to ages 22–39.
[c] Number of cases based only on the women who want no more children.
[d] Frequency is weighted as follows: urban respondents × 4 and rural respondents × 12.

Table 2.5 (Continued)

Wife's age (years) and number of living children	Philippines 1968	Taiwan 1967	Taiwan[b] 1970	Thailand (urban) 1970	Thailand (rural) 1969	Belgium 1966	Great Britain 1967–68	Hungary 1966	United States 1965
20–24	88	74	46	60	90	20	17	18	33
25–29	82	53	45	44	86	7	7	18	22
30–34	80	47	33	33	86	8	6	19	17
35–39	84	43	33	44	89	14	10	27	19
Total	83	47	36	41	88	12	8	22	21
20–29	84	56	45	49	87	10	9	18	26
<2 children	88	77	0	50	92	11	0	16	61
2	88	58	42	62	88	7	10	16	20
3	81	54	48	53	88	4	11	24	25
4	80	57	39	38	81	21	—	—	19
5 or more	86	53	50	33	—	—	—	—	22
30–39	82	45	33	39	88	12	8	21	18
<2 children	85	73	57	70	71	20	6	25	41
2	82	33	42	37	94	8	6	17	14
3	80	40	26	27	86	9	6	19	11
4	79	40	32	42	92	8	16	32	14
5 or more	83	50	35	41	87	6	21	39	20
20–39	83	47	36	41	88	12	8	20	21
<2 children	87	73	57	57	84	18	5	21	47
2	86	48	42	48	90	8	7	17	16
3	81	46	35	36	87	8	7	20	16
4	80	43	33	41	88	9	17	35	16
5 or more	83	50	37	40	87	7	19	40	20
Number of Cases[c]	14,740[d]	2,313	1,521	543	370	1,728	632	3,791	2,316

2 to 31 percent practice contraception, while in the developed countries 62 to 68 percent do so. For age group 35–39, the two ranges are 12 to 50 percent and 69 to 77 percent.

In the developed countries, since the percentage practicing contraception at the youngest ages is so large, the age gradient is not very steep. The proportions practicing contraception at the older ages are not as high as one might expect, probably because more older women know they are subfecund and because some (especially in Hungary) are relying on abortion.

In the developing countries only a few populations have a steep age gradient in the practice of contraception. Taiwan and Korea, for example, both had active population programs and considerable individual practice of contraception without program assistance at the time of their surveys. By ages 30–34 and 35–39, there are, therefore, much higher rates of contraceptive use in Taiwan and Korea than, for example, in India and West Malaysia.

Given these facts, it is not surprising that at every age the proportion not currently practicing contraception among those who want no more children is: (1) moderately large to very large in all the developing populations, and (2) much greater in the developing than in the developed populations (Table 2.5). In India, Jakarta, Korea, Mexico City, West Malaysia, rural East Java, and rural Thailand, in almost every age group a majority, and usually a very large majority, of those who report that they want no more children are not practicing contraception. In Taiwan, Korea, and Ankara, the proportion decreases considerably with age; even so, in these populations the percentage of nonpractice among those who want no more children is between 43 and 61 percent at ages 30–34 and 35–39. Delhi is the one developing population in which the percentage of nonusers among those wanting no more children is less than 50 percent in all age groups.

The discrepant group, those who want no more children and yet are not practicing contraception, increases rapidly with age in most of the developing populations (Table 2.6), because for most countries the desire for no more children increases faster than the practice of contraception among such couples. Hence, by age 35–39 the proportion of people in the discrepant situation ranges from 24 to 66 percent in the developing populations and from 9 to 24 percent in the developed populations (the high figure of 24 percent for Hungary results from the reliance on abortion by many older women). In each age group the size of the discrepant group depends, of course, on the level of the two components that determine it, as we have already illustrated for four countries in Table 2.2.

Variations by Parity

Parity has a different relation to the two components in developed and developing countries (Tables 2.3 and 2.5). Therefore, the two groups of countries differ in the relation of parity to the proportions who want no more children and are not practicing contraception (Tables 2.6 and 2.7).

In the developed countries there is relatively little variation with parity (after the first child) in the proportions who want no more and are not practicing contraception. At all parities after the first, a majority of women in the developed countries want no more children (Table 2.3) and among them the majority use contraception (Table 2.5). Again, the apparent exception for Hungary is explained by considerable reliance there on induced abortion, especially at the higher parities. The proportions in the discrepant group reach 14 to 18 percent in both Great Britain and the United States at the fourth and fifth parities, but this involves relatively small numbers of women, especially in Great Britain.

The situation is quite different and more varied in the developing countries. There, the relative size of the discrepant group increases quite rapidly with parity; as with age, this reflects more rapid increase in the proportions wanting no more children than in the proportions practicing contraception (Tables 2.3 through 2.5). The considerable variations among the developing countries result from the fact that: (1) in some populations, such as Mexico and West Malaysia, women want large families and, therefore, relatively few want no more children until they reach the fourth and fifth parities; and (2) in some other populations, such as Delhi, urban Thailand, and Taiwan in 1970, many women have adopted contraception to prevent unwanted births at moderate parities (for example, at the third and fourth parities).

Despite these variations among countries, at every parity after the first, the relative size of the discrepant group is greater for any of the developing countries than for any of the developed countries, apart from Hungary, which is strongly affected by abortion. The only exceptions are second and third parity women in Mexico City; few of them want no more children.

In some populations (India, Jakarta, West Malaysia, the Philippines, and rural Thailand) at every parity for either younger or older women, a large majority of those who want no more children are not practicing contraception. Since the proportion who want no more children increases with parity in these places, the result is that at higher parities (for example, four

Table 2.6 Percentage Who Want No More Children and Are Not Using Contraception, by Wife's Age and Number of Living Children, for Married Women Aged 20–39 Years

Wife's age (years) and number of living children	Ankara[a] 1966	Calcutta 1970	Delhi 1968–69	India 1970	Rural East Java 1972	Jakarta 1968	Korea 1971	West Malaysia 1966–67	Mexico City 1971
20–24	26	13	9	20	5	17	7	11	12
25–29	36	20	14	35	19	30	18	18	31
30–34	28	30	18	50	27	57	35	28	44
35–39	37	42	24	58	43	54	48	44	50
Total	32	26	16	41	24	38	30	25	35
20–29	32	17	12	28	13	25	14	15	23
<2 children	4	3	4	8	5	8	4	3	0
2	32	14	22	28	12	18	19	11	0
3	39	31	29	46	15	33	28	18	9
4	71	42	22	70	22	54	23	35	23
5 or more	—	—	33	54	27	54	—	43	63
30–39	32	36	21	54	34	53	42	34	47
<2 children	2	15	30	21	24	27	16	12	—
2	23	30	11	37	32	44	36	14	—
3	36	34	15	56	35	61	34	21	1
4	33	47	17	70	42	61	39	34	23
5 or more	67	50	—	68	36	71	54	48	68
20–39	32	26	16	41	24	38	30	25	35
<2 children	3	7	9	11	12	15	6	5	0
2	28	20	15	31	18	26	25	12	0
3	37	33	20	51	22	41	32	19	6
4	46	45	19	70	33	58	37	34	23
5 or more	72	50	24	66	35	67	54	47	67
Number of Cases	552	947	5,242	10,246	1,418	811	1,622	4,242	486

NOTE: See Appendix 1, item 3 for definitions. Sterilization included as contraception except in Belgium and Great Britain.
— = Less than 20 cases in the category.
[a] Defined as "percent wanting no more children and never used contraception."
[b] Taiwan 1970 data refer to ages 22–39.
[c] Frequency is weighted as follows: urban respondents × 4 and rural respondents × 12.

Table 2.6 (Continued)

Wife's age (years) and number of living children	Philippines 1968	Taiwan 1967	Taiwan[b] 1970	Thailand (urban) 1970	Thailand (rural) 1969	Belgium 1966	Great Britain 1967-68	Hungary 1966	United States 1965
20-24	18	7	6	14	28	6	3	5	11
25-29	34	19	17	17	39	3	3	10	12
30-34	46	33	26	19	52	6	4	15	13
35-39	60	37	30	31	66	12	9	24	16
Total	42	25	22	21	50	8	5	14	13
20-29	28	14	14	16	35	4	3	9	12
<2 children	7	0	0	5	14	3	0	5	8
2	22	11	8	19	36	5	6	13	10
3	32	24	24	28	48	3	9	21	17
4	48	40	26	29	50	15	—	40	14
5 or more	66	46	42	30	—	—	—	—	19
30-39	53	35	28	24	60	10	6	19	14
<2 children	11	16	21	9	12	14	4	18	24
2	31	14	24	17	43	7	5	16	11
3	35	26	20	16	53	7	5	18	9
4	49	33	28	32	62	7	14	29	13
5 or more	69	46	33	34	73	5	18	34	18
20-39	42	25	22	21	50	8	5	14	13
<2 children	8	2	3	6	14	10	1	10	14
2	25	12	12	18	38	6	5	15	11
3	33	25	22	20	51	6	6	19	12
4	48	35	27	32	58	8	14	31	14
5 or more	68	46	34	33	72	6	17	34	18
Number of Cases	28,964[c]	4,300	2,491	1,080	642	2,567	1,088	5,309	3,593

Table 2.7 Range in Percentage Wanting No More Children and Not Using Contraception, by Number of Living Children, for Developing and Developed Countries

Number of living children	Developing countries	Three developed countries[a]
2	0–38[b]	5–11
3	6–51[c]	6–12
4	19–70	8–14
5 or more	33–70	6–18

[a] Hungary omitted because reliance on abortion results in high proportions at higher parities.
[b] Range 12–38 if Mexico City is excluded.
[c] Range 20–51 if Mexico City is excluded.

and five or more) as many as 40 to 70 percent of all women say they want no more children but are not practicing contraception.

In another group of developing populations (Taiwan, Korea, urban Thailand, and Delhi), the proportions who want no more but are not practicing contraception are not only smaller but tend to decrease with parity. Therefore, in these countries in the important parities from three onward, the proportions in the discrepant group are in the lower range for developing countries, although they are substantially greater than for developed countries.

It is important to remember that, as compared with the developed countries, much larger proportions of couples in the developing countries are in the higher parities where the discrepant groups are largest. Although this makes the total size of the discrepant group larger, since age and parity go together, it also means that the potential for reducing fertility in the long run is less than it would be if more of the younger and lower parity women wanted no more children. Still, in most developing countries a large proportion of births are to women over age 30 and at higher parities.[4] The large reduction in fertility in such places as Taiwan in the last decade was among just such high parity older women.

Among women at the same parity, the relation of age to the relative size of the discrepant group varies among developing countries. In some developing populations it is always greater for older women (30–39)

---

[4] United Nations, *The Determinants and Consequences of Population Trends* (New York: United Nations, 1973), Chapter IV.

than for younger women (20–29) (Calcutta, West Malaysia, the Philippines, East Java, Jakarta); but in others the reverse is true at some parities (India, West Malaysia); and in still others the reverse is true at most parities (Ankara, Delhi, Mexico City).

These differing patterns result from the nature of the balance between completely opposite trends by age within parity for the two components. Almost always—in 35 of 43 comparisons by age within parity—the proportion who want no more children is greater for older than for younger women at specific parities (Table 2.3). Usually (43 of 57 comparisons) the proportion practicing contraception among those wanting no more children is greater for younger than for older women at specific parities (Table 2.5). The size of the discrepant group for younger and older women at a particular parity depends on the balance between the two opposite forces: (1) fewer younger women at any parity want no more children, but (2) among this smaller number a larger proportion practice contraception. The situation in any particular developing country requires an assessment of the differing levels of the two components.

Educational Differentials

Wife's education was selected as the major modernization variable in this analysis, since it has been found to be an important correlate of fertility in many studies. The discussion, again, is based mainly on data for women over age 30, since both education and the demographic measures are strongly dependent on age at marriage at younger ages and the samples of the younger ages variably represent those who will marry later.

Broadly speaking, in the developing countries the proportion of wives over age 30 who say that they want no more children is high in all educational strata (except in West Malaysia) and does not vary systematically with education (Table 2.8). On the other hand, every developing population shows a marked positive association between education and the practice of contraception, both for all couples and for those who want no more children (Tables 2.9 and 2.10). The net result is that the discrepant behavior group tends to decrease with education in every developing country considered (Table 2.11).

These differentials by education within countries do not mean that women of similar educational levels are even roughly comparable in different developing countries, either with respect to the use of contraception among those who want no more children or in the relative size of the

Table 2.8 Percentage Wanting No More Children, by Wife's Age and Education, for Married Women Aged 20–39 Years

Wife's age (years) and education	Ankara 1966	Calcutta 1970	India 1970	Korea 1971	West Malaysia 1966–67	West Malaysia 1970	Mexico City 1971	Philippines 1968	Taiwan 1967	Taiwan[a] 1970	Thailand (urban) 1970	Thailand (rural) 1969
20–29												
No formal	50	36	35	19	17	17	34	37	26	32	32	40
Primary	57	36	33	32	18	19	36	21	29	38	36	54
Junior high	52	42	40	16	18	17	38	40	24	29	33	37
Senior high and over	36	43	*	21	10	14	29	39	29	37	39	—
	29	27	42	16	8	7	—	33	19	25	14	—
30–39												
No formal	62	72	67	72	43	36	63	66	78	84	62	68
Primary	65	71	64	72	43	34	69	50	77	84	68	66
Junior high	66	91	79	72	43	38	64	69	78	85	64	69
Senior high and over	64	85	*	73	38	36	55	74	82	82	64	—
	38	60	81	71	36	35	—	61	76	79	40	—
20–39												
No formal	56	54	51	50	31	26	48	54	54	61	50	58
Primary	61	55	49	63	34	29	53	39	56	67	62	63
Junior high	58	66	58	47	28	26	51	56	53	59	51	57
Senior high and over	53	62	*	47	22	21	40	58	54	58	52	—
	34	43	58	41	19	17	33	51	44	48	28	—
Number of Cases	552	947	10,246	1,620	4,242	13,449	486	25,604[b]	4,300	2,491	1,080	642

NOTE: See Appendix 1, items 3 and 6 for definitions.
— = Less than 20 cases in the category.
* = No such category.

[a] Taiwan 1970 data refer to ages 22–39.
[b] Frequency is weighted as follows: urban respondents × 4 and rural respondents × 12.

Table 2.9 Percentage Currently Using Contraception, by Wife's Age and Education, for Married Women Aged 20–39 Years

Wife's age (years) and education	Ankara[a] 1966	Calcutta 1970	India 1970	Korea 1971	West Malaysia 1966-67	West Malaysia 1970	Mexico City 1971	Philippines 1968	Taiwan 1967	Taiwan[b] 1970	Thailand (urban) 1970	Thailand (rural) 1969
20–29	42	38	10	10	7	17	23	16	16	26	34	9
No formal	18	18	5	12	2	11	2	9	12	21	18	0
Primary	38	38	18	10	7	17	20	14	16	22	33	10
Junior high	41	37	*	6	12	26	41	20	26	48	43	—
Senior high and over	68	65	30	14	33	30	—	29	36	49	37	—
30–39	41	43	15	33	11	19	25	18	45	58	48	16
No formal	26	23	10	22	5	13	8	11	37	51	33	9
Primary	50	51	21	36	17	23	21	15	48	61	50	17
Junior high	61	60	*	41	36	36	51	22	66	72	57	—
Senior high and over	62	66	46	39	49	47	—	34	70	81	55	—
20–39	37	40	12	24	9	18	24	17	32	44	42	13
No formal	22	21	8	20	4	12	5	10	26	39	30	6
Primary	43	44	19	24	11	19	21	15	33	43	43	14
Junior high	53	47	*	24	23	29	45	21	45	60	50	—
Senior high and over	65	65	36	26	39	36	47	32	51	63	47	—
Number of Cases	552	947	10,246	1,620	4,242	13,449	486	25,604[c]	4,300	2,491	1,080	642

NOTE: See Appendix 1, item 6 for definitions. Sterilization included as contraception except in Belgium and Great Britain.
— = Less than 20 cases in the category.
* = No such category.

[a] Defined as "ever used contraception."
[b] Taiwan 1970 data refer to ages 22–39.
[c] Frequency is weighted as follows: urban respondents × 4 and rural respondents × 12.

Table 2.10 Of Those Who Want No More Children, Percentage Not Using Contraception, by Wife's Age and Education, for Married Women Aged 20-39 Years

Wife's age (years) and education	Ankara[a] 1966	Calcutta 1970	Delhi 1968-69	India 1970	Jakarta 1968	Korea 1971	West Malaysia 1966-67	Mexico City 1971	Philippines 1968	Taiwan 1967	Taiwan[b] 1970	Thailand (urban) 1970	Thailand (rural) 1969
20-29													
No formal	64	48	33	80	89	73	87	68	84	56	45	49	87
Primary	79	59	56	89	100	78	92	—	95	63	53	—	—
Junior high	53	—	23	67	92	66	87	73	87	56	48	51	86
Senior high and over	—	52	15	*	78	85	—	—	74	39	16	45	—
	—	26	12	54	67	—	—	—	69	28	11	—	—
30-39													
No formal	53	49	27	80	89	58	80	75	82	45	33	39	88
Primary	65	68	44	85	95	72	89	92	96	54	42	54	94
Junior high	45	44	19	77	89	53	72	77	85	42	31	36	87
Senior high and over	38	37	10	*	89	47	43	44	76	26	17	31	—
	—	23	7	46	45	45	32	—	62	21	6	30	—
20-39													
No formal	58	49	29	80	89	60	82	72	83	47	36	41	88
Primary	71	65	48	86	97	73	89	93	95	56	44	56	96
Junior high	49	45	20	73	91	55	77	75	86	45	35	40	87
Senior high and over	41	43	11	*	80	56	54	39	75	30	17	36	—
	23	26	9	49	61	52	37	—	64	23	8	23	—
Number of Cases[c]	310	511	3,009	5,195	367	795	1,302	234	13,776[d]	2,313	1,521	543	370

NOTE: See Appendix 1, items 3 and 6 for definitions. Sterilization included as contraception except in Belgium and Great Britain.
— = Less than 20 cases in the category.
* = No such category.
[a] Defined as "of those wanting no more children, percent never used contraception."
[b] Taiwan 1970 data refer to ages 22-39.
[c] Number of cases based only on the women who want no more children.
[d] Frequency is weighted as follows: urban respondents × 4 and rural respondents × 12.

Table 2.11 Percentage Who Want No More Children and Are Not Using Contraception, by Wife's Age and Education, for Married Women Aged 20–39 Years

Wife's age (years) and education	Ankara[a] 1966	Calcutta 1970	Delhi 1968–69	India 1970	Jakarta 1968	Korea 1971	West Malaysia 1966–67	Mexico City 1971	Philippines 1968	Taiwan 1967	Taiwan[b] 1970	Thailand (urban) 1970	Thailand (rural) 1969
20–29	32	17	12	28	25	14	15	23	31	14	14	16	35
No formal	45	21	48	29	35	25	16	35	20	18	20	25	54
Primary	27	20	12	26	26	11	16	27	35	13	14	17	32
Junior high	18	22	7	*	18	18	8	9	29	11	6	18	—
Senior high and over	6	7	4	22	2	12	4	—	22	5	3	0	—
30–39	32	36	21	54	53	42	34	47	54	35	28	24	60
No formal	42	48	50	55	64	52	38	63	48	41	35	37	62
Primary	30	40	13	61	53	38	31	50	59	33	26	24	60
Junior high	24	32	5	*	34	34	16	24	56	21	14	20	—
Senior high and over	9	14	6	37	10	32	12	—	38	16	4	12	—
20–39	32	26	16	41	38	30	25	35	44	25	22	21	50
No formal	44	36	49	42	53	46	31	49	38	31	30	34	60
Primary	29	30	12	43	36	26	22	38	48	24	20	21	49
Junior high	22	27	6	*	23	26	12	15	43	16	10	18	—
Senior high and over	8	10	4	28	5	22	7	13	32	10	4	6	—
Number of Cases	552	947	5,242	10,246	811	1,620	4,242	486	25,604[c]	4,300	2,491	1,080	642

NOTE: See Appendix 1, items 3 and 6 for definitions. Sterilization included as contraception except in Belgium and Great Britain.
— = Less than 20 cases in the category.
* = No such category.

[a] Defined as "percent wanting no more children and never used contraception."
[b] Taiwan 1970 data refer to ages 22–39.
[c] Frequency is weighted as follows: urban respondents × 4 and rural respondents × 12.

discrepant group. For example, among women with senior high school education who want no more children, the proportion not practicing contraception is very low in Delhi and Taiwan (7 to 21 percent), moderately high in Korea and India (45 to 46 percent), and very high in the Philippines (62 percent). Women in the most educated stratum in the Philippines had a higher proportion not practicing contraception than women without any education in Taiwan and urban Thailand.

In the lowest educational stratum (those with no education, which includes many of the women in developing countries) the proportions not practicing contraception among those who want no more children are very high—85 to 95 percent—in some places (India, Jakarta, West Malaysia, Mexico City, the Philippines, rural Thailand). The proportions are considerably lower—42 to 72 percent—in other populations where the general level of contraceptive practice is higher (Calcutta, Delhi, Korea, Taiwan, urban Thailand).

In the developed countries at age 30–39, the percentage wanting no more children is high at all educational levels and does not vary systematically with education, except in Belgium where with more education there is a moderate decrease in the percentage wanting no more children (Table 2.12). The proportion who are not practicing contraception among those who want no more children and the percentage who are not practicing *and* want no more children decrease systematically with education for each of the four developed populations. However, for those women who consider their childbearing completed, both the levels of nonpractice and the amount of variation with education are very small in Belgium and Great Britain. The greater variation with education in Hungary is a result of greater reliance on abortion among the less educated. In the United States the levels of current nonpractice among women who want no more children are also relatively high, particularly among those who have less than a high school education.

Among those who want no more children, even the best-educated women in most developing countries are less likely to be practicing contraception than the least-educated women in the developed countries (compare Tables 2.10 and 2.12). This is true for India, Korea, Jakarta, and the Philippines. In a few developing populations (Taiwan, Calcutta, Delhi) the women at the higher educational levels are more likely to be practicing contraception than are more poorly educated women in the United States and Hungary.

Insofar as education is an index of modernization, its effect on individuals appears to be related to what is happening in the country as a whole.

In countries such as Taiwan and Korea and in some of the urban centers of the developing countries, even among women without education, significant proportions are reporting practice of contraception when no more children are wanted. On the other hand, in other developing countries where contraceptive use is generally low, even well-educated women are still making relatively little use of contraceptives.

On the Validity and Reliability of the Data

Why do so many couples in the developing countries who say that they want no more children fail to practice contraception? One possible explanation is that the measures about wanting children are grossly defective. It has been argued that the respondents in developing countries give the interviewers the answers that are expected—biased toward smaller families than they really want. Another line of argument is that the attitude statements must be invalid or very low in salience because, if the couples really wanted no more children, they would be sufficiently motivated to adopt contraception from commercial or official program sources or to use such methods as withdrawal or abortion.[5]

It is undoubtedly true that the category, "wanting no more children," must include respondents whose attitudes vary greatly in salience, intensity, and validity. Reinterviews might result in shifting a significant number of responses from "want no more" to "want more" or "uncertain" or "up to God," although we do not know that this would occur. But, the proposition that what people say they want should be rejected out-of-hand cannot be accepted on the basis of a verbal assumption of a lack of credibility. Certainly, the fact that the discrepancy between attitude and behavior exists is not proof that the statements are invalid.

Attitudes and behavior often are inconsistent, especially in a time of rapid social change when not all aspects of society can be expected to change at the same pace. The IUSSP project included time series data from Taiwan that are pertinent to the issue of a time lag between attitude and behavior. As Table 2.13 indicates, in 1965, 48 percent of the Taiwanese women aged 30–39 wanted no more children and were not practicing contraception. Taking only that single cross-section survey, one might argue

---

[5] For example, see P. M. Hauser, "Family planning programs: A book review article," *Demography* 4, no. 1 (1967): 397–414; K. Davis, "Population policy: Will current programs succeed?" *Science,* 158 (November 1967): 730–739.

Table 2.12 Percentage Wanting No More Children and Contraceptive Status by Wife's Age and Education, for Married Women Aged 20–39 Years, for Four Developed Countries

Wife's age (years) and education	United States 1970	Hungary 1966	Belgium 1966	Great Britain 1967–68	United States 1970	Hungary 1966	Belgium 1966	Great Britain 1967–68
	Percent wanting no more children				Percent not using contraception among those who want no more			
20–29								
Less than high school	46	44	42	34	25	18	10	9
Some high school	65	46	47	36[a]	28	20	11	9
High school graduate and over	60	38	40	31[a]	28	9	9	9
	41	29	28		24	12	3	
30–39								
Less than high school	88	84	79	82	21	23	12	8
Some high school	89	83	81	82	25	25	13	
High school graduate and over	89	86	78	81	26	16	10	10
	88	74	69		19	13	11	4
20–39								
Less than high school	65	66	67	58	22	22	12	8
Some high school	80	68	72	60	26	23	12	
High school graduate and over	74	59	64	54	27	13	10	10
	62	57	53		21	12	10	6

Table 2.12 (continued)

Wife's age (years) and education	United States 1970	Hungary 1966	Belgium 1966	Great Britain 1967–68	United States 1970	Hungary 1966	Belgium 1966	Great Britain 1967–68
	Percent currently using contraception				Percent who want no more children and are not using contraception			
20–29								
Less than high school	68	68	74	69	11	8	4	3
Some high school	64	66	75	67	18	9	5	3
High school graduate and over	65	73	73	72	17	3	4	3
	68	72	72		10	3	2	
30–39								
Less than high school	75	70	76	75	18	20	10	6
Some high school	71	69	75	73	22	21	10	8
High school graduate and over	70	79	80	80	23	13	8	3
	77	76	79		17	9	8	
20–39								
Less than high school	71	69	76	72	14	14	8	5
Some high school	68	68	75	70	21	16	9	6
High school graduate and over	67	76	77	76	20	8	7	3
	72	75	76		13	7	5	
Total Number of Cases	4,724	5,937	2,567	1,088				

[a] For Great Britain the two educational groups are those who terminated education under age 16 and at age 16 or older. See Appendix 1, item 7 for other definitional variations.

Table 2.13 Trend for 1965–1970 in Attitudes About Number of Children and Use of Contraception, Taiwan, Married Women, Aged 30–39 Years

Item	1965	1967	1970
Percent who want no more children	79	78	84
Percent currently using contraception	38	55	72
Percent who are not using contraception among those who want no more children	60	45	33
Percent who want no more children and are not using contraception	48	35	28
Mean ideal number of children	4.2	4.0	3.9

that with so many discrepant cases, many of the statements about wanting no more children are simply invalid. However, the trend data show that during the following five-year period, when there was relatively little change in the proportion who wanted no more or in their mean ideal number of children, there was a very substantial increase in the practice of contraception by those who wanted no more children, so that there was a large reduction in the proportion of discrepant cases.

A plausible interpretation of these results (developed in detail elsewhere[6]) is that with little change in long-standing values about desired number of children, contraception was adopted rapidly to reduce the number of unwanted children that were being born because of prior declines in mortality. It is plausible that in 1965 many women had a problem—they wanted no more children—but it took some time for them to perceive that contraception was a safe, legitimate, feasible way to solve this problem. If this was the case in Taiwan, it might well be true in other developing countries as well. A time lag between having a goal and acting to achieve it is plausible. The existence of the discrepant group is not in itself conclusive evidence that the measurement of the attitude is invalid.

Another consideration is that whether a particular attitude will lead to appropriate behavior will depend on a constellation of related attitudes. For example, we have seen that in some of the IUSSP surveys respondents who already had the number of children they considered ideal nevertheless said they wanted more and were not using contraception, presumably because they did not have the number of sons considered important in that

---

[6] R. Freedman, L. C. Coombs, and M.-C. Chang, "Trends in family size preferences and practice of family planning: Taiwan, 1965–1970," *Studies in Family Planning* 3, no. 12 (December 1972): 281–296.

society. Apparently in such places as Taiwan and Korea, couples are prepared to have more children than they consider desirable if that is necessary to have the one or two sons they consider essential. In an unpublished longitudinal follow-up study in Taiwan, it was found that those who had more children, although they previously said they wanted no more, initially had no sons or only one.[7] In addition to the preference for sons, there must be other attitudes that should be taken into account when viewing apparently discrepant behavior.

To some extent, the discrepancy may simply reflect fecundity impairments. Some women who do not want more children are not using contraception because they are subfecund and, therefore, unlikely to become pregnant. In such countries as the United States, Belgium, and Great Britain, the percentage who are not practicing contraception when they want no more children is low enough to make this a plausible explanation for many of the discrepant cases. There is confirming evidence that this is a major explanation for nonuse of contraception in later stages of family life in the United States.[8] But in most of the developing populations, the level of the discrepancy is much too large to be explained by any plausible estimate of subfecundity. For Taiwan, for example, if the subfecund are omitted, then among women aged 20–39 the percent who want no more children and are not practicing contraception is only reduced from 25 to 21 percent.

The IUSSP group, which discussed the comparative data in a seminar, agreed that answers to a single question—"do you want more children?" or "how many children do you consider ideal for your family?"—are likely to be unreliable for at least some and perhaps for many respondents. But the real issue is: How unreliable, for how many, and in what kinds of situations? Given the scientific and practical importance of the discrepancy phenomenon, the IUSSP group agreed that it would be unwise simply to dismiss the phenomenon as a methodological artifact on the basis of an assertion of lack of validity. Instead, the group endorsed the desirability of the following kinds of empirical work to increase our knowledge of what the discrepancy means:

1. Establish time series, such as those illustrated for Taiwan, as a basis for plausible inferences about changes in the components making up the discrepancy.

---

[7] Unpublished analysis by R. Freedman, from the third Taiwan KAP study, consisting of a follow-up of women interviewed in 1967.
[8] For example, see P. K. Whelpton, A. A. Campbell, and J. E. Patterson, *Fertility and Family Planning in the United States* (Princeton: Princeton University Press, 1966).

2. Conduct longitudinal studies to find out what happens to the contraceptive practice, fertility desires, and fertility performance of the discrepant and nondiscrepant cases over a period of time. Wherever possible, link such longitudinal studies to action programs to see whether those who say they want no more children adopt contraception if it is offered by a well-organized family planning program.

3. Use skilled interviewers and systematic participant observation to try to establish for matched samples of discrepant and nondiscrepant cases whether the attitude statement was stable and, if so, why contraception was not being used.

4. Encourage the use and assessment of several measures of desired family size and sex preference that might reflect different aspects of the basic attitude complex. Encourage the development of more rational and sensitive measures that may involve using a series of questions designed in advance to be tested for internal consistency by psychological and logical principles.

5. Do everything possible to improve the control over the quality of field work, concentrating on questions that have been tested on a comparative basis. This is a major goal of the World Fertility Survey, which was just being organized as the IUSSP subcommittee completed its work.

Appendix ONE

Summary Notes on Definitions

For each of the variables discussed, the standard definition used in the majority of countries is stated, followed by the variations. Categories of education and urban-rural residence are described.

1. Ideal Number of Sons. Standard definition: number of sons wanted if the respondent could start over.

Calcutta: defined as a generalized ideal.

India: defined as the number of living sons plus the number of additional sons desired.

Korea: defined as a generalized ideal.

West Malaysia (1966–67): for women who said they wanted more children, defined as the number of living sons plus the number of additional sons desired; for women who said they wanted no more or were uncertain, defined as a personal ideal if the respondent could start over.

Hungary: defined as the number of living sons plus the number of additional sons desired.

United States: defined as a generalized ideal.

For the number and handling of indeterminate responses on this variable (and on ideal number of children and additional children wanted) see the Introduction section on "Methodological Problems" and Appendix 2.

2. Ideal Number of Children. Standard definition: number of children wanted if the respondent could start over.

Calcutta: defined as a generalized ideal.

India: defined as a generalized ideal.

Korea: defined as a generalized ideal.

West Malaysia (1966–67): where compared to ideal number of sons, ideal number of children is defined as follows: for women who said they wanted more children, it is the number of living children plus the number of additional children desired; for women who said they wanted no more or were uncertain, it is defined as a personal ideal if the respondent could start over. In tables involving only ideal number of children, it is defined as a generalized ideal.

Hungary: where compared with ideal number of sons, defined as the number of living children plus the number of additional children desired.

Great Britain: defined as the numerical answer to a complex question about the number of children the respondent really wanted in relation to the number she expected.

United States: defined as a generalized ideal, except in Table 1.7 where it is defined as the desired number of children.

3. Wanting No More Children. Standard definition: no additional children wanted in answer to the question, "How many (more) children do you want?"

Ankara: defined as present parity greater than or equal to ideal (if respondent could start over).

Calcutta: women indifferent to wanting more (12.7 percent) are not classified as wanting no more.

West Malaysia (1970): defined as present parity greater than or equal to ideal (if respondent could start over).

Mexico City: defined as present parity greater than or equal to ideal (if respondent could start over).

Belgium: defined as present parity greater than or equal to total number of children expected.

Great Britain: defined as expect no more.

United States: defined as intend no more.

4. Number of Additional Children Wanted. Standard definition: the answer to question, "How many (more) children do you want?"

Ankara: defined as the number wanted (a personal ideal) minus the number of living children.

Calcutta: defined as total number of children desired minus the number of living children (if woman desires more).

Mexico City: defined as the number wanted (a personal ideal) minus the number of living children.

Belgium: defined as the total number expected minus the number of living children.

Great Britain: defined as the number of additional children expected.

United States: defined as the number of additional children intended.

5. Expect More Than Ideal. Standard definition: when the woman wants or expects more children than her ideal (if she could start over).

Calcutta: defined as when the number of living children or total number of children desired is greater than ideal (a generalized ideal).
India: defined as want more than ideal (a generalized ideal).
Korea: defined as want more than ideal (a generalized ideal).
United States: defined as intend more than ideal.

6. **Educational Categories in Developing Countries.** For cross-country comparability some categories of education were combined as follows:

Calcutta: Junior high = secondary; senior high and over = some higher secondary, completed high school, pre-university and above, combined.
Delhi: No formal = illiterate and no formal combined.
India: Senior high and over = secondary and college combined.
Jakarta: Senior high and over = senior high and over combined.
West Malaysia (1970): No formal = no schooling and other (nonformal) education combined; primary = some years primary and completed primary, combined; junior high = Form I to III; senior high and over = Form IV and above.
Philippines: Primary = grades 1–4 and grades 5–7 combined; junior high = high school 1–3; senior high and over = high school graduate, college 1–3 and college graduate combined.
Thailand (urban): Primary = primary 1–4 and primary 5–7 combined.
Thailand (rural): Primary = primary 1–4.

7. **Educational Categories in Developed Countries.** Because the important education levels differ in the developed and the developing countries, a separate table (Table 2.12) based on different broad levels is presented. Some categories of education were combined to form levels as follows:

United States: Less than high school = grade school 0–8; some high school = high school 1–3; high school graduate and over = high school 4 and college combined.
Hungary: Less than high school = women not having attended at school and primary (1–8 classes) combined; some high school = junior high (8–12); high school graduate and over = senior high and over (13+).
Belgium: Less than high school = primary; some high school = junior high; high school graduate and over = senior high and over.

8. **Urban-Rural Residence Categories.** Where categories of urban-rural residence shown here are different from the categories used in the studies, the equivalents are as follows:

India: Large city = urban 500,000 population and over; small city = urban 100,000–500,000 population; urban township = other urban; rural township = rural.

Korea: Large city = Seoul and industrial cities combined; small city = other city; urban township = rural township; rural township = rural.

West Malaysia (1966–67): Large city = metropolis; small city = small town; rural township = rural.

West Malaysia (1970): Large city = metropolitan towns; small city = towns; rural township = rural areas.

Philippines: Large city = urban 20,000 population and over; small city = urban less than 20,000 population; urban township = rural 20,000 population and over; rural township = rural less than 20,000 population.

United States: Large city = central city of Standard Metropolitan Statistical Area (SMSA) and ring of SMSA combined; small city = cities less than 50,000 population; urban township = rural nonfarm; rural township = rural farm.

Appendix T W O

Methodological Statements for the Individual Studies

Each investigator prepared a statement about such methodological issues as sample size and design and the definitions and procedures pertinent to the specific variables used in the study. An effort was made to keep these brief, and the topics to be included were specified by the conference participants. The information about definitions for all the material presented in this comparative report has been incorporated into Appendix 1. Some further definitional detail on variables not used here is available in the IUSSP files. At the request of the conference of investigators, information on the other methodological topics is reproduced here so that the reader will be aware of the variations among the investigations and be able to view methodological problems in light of the basic materials.

ANKARA

A. Specification of sample

1. Size: There were a total of 803 interviews.

2. Universe sampled and frame used: The universe sampled was currently married women living in Ankara. The political definition of Ankara corresponds to something between an urbanized area and a Standard Metropolitan Statistical Area (SMSA) in US census terminology. The frame for the sample was the listing of all households in Ankara developed for the census of 1965 only a few months prior to the study. There were approximately 170,000 households in Ankara at the time. The household list was subdivided into chunks of 100 households (combinations or portions of blocks) and stratified by the economic characteristics of the chunks (impressions of the staff of the Turkish State Institute of Statistics of the status of each chunk—slum or non-slum). A systematic sample of one out of every eight chunks was selected, yielding about 210 chunks. Within each selected chunk, four households were selected systematically.

3. *Primary respondents:* Currently married women.

4. *Identification and weighting:* This design produces an equal probability of selection for each household. If more than one couple lived in the household, a printed random selection on the schedule determined which wife was to be interviewed.

5. *Response rate:* Interviews were completed in nearly 99 percent of the selected eligible households.

B. *Handling of indeterminates*

Interviewers were sent back to the households if questions were skipped or missed. At several places in the interview where we anticipated some resistance or ambiguity of response (for example, expected number of additional children), a series of probes were written into the schedule to convert initially ambiguous responses to numerical responses. The latter were used in all the tables presented. For the remaining one or two percent NAs (not ascertained), random, or internal consistency procedures were used, depending on the particular question involved. In the data presented here, the small number of NAs were eliminated completely. Given the small number of NAs, any procedure used could not have affected the overall results.

C. *Prevalence of induced abortion*

After obtaining a live birth history, the respondent was asked: "Did you ever have any pregnancies that did not result in a live birth? For instance, stillbirths, miscarriages, or abortions. How many? How did the (1st, 2nd, etc.) pregnancy end? Was it a stillbirth, miscarriage, or abortion?" About 20 percent of the women reported an abortion.

D. *Prevalence of divorce and remarriage*

About 6 percent of the women reported more than one marriage.

BELGIUM

A. *Specification of sample*

1. *Size:* 3,022 usable questionnaires.

2. *Universe sampled and frame used:* National.

3. *Primary respondents:* Married women; aged 40 years or less; husband present.

4. *Identification and weighting:* Probability proportional to size.

5. *Response rate:* No information.

B. *Handling of indeterminates*

NAs excluded in calculations of means, but included in calculations of percentages.

C. **Prevalence of induced abortion**

No data available.

D. **Prevalence of divorce and remarriage**

49 remarriages among respondents.

CALCUTTA

A. **Specification of sample**

1. Size: 947 married women in the age group 20–39 years, comprising one subsample only, formed the basis of present tabulations. The total sample consisted of four such subsamples.

2. Universe sampled and frame used: About 6,000 sample households from 304 blocks selected from 3,872 blocks in the Municipal Corporation Area of Calcutta. Two blocks were excluded at the outset because they consisted of military barracks only. The sampling frame consisting of blocks was provided by the Urban Frame Survey of the National Sample Survey.

3. Primary respondents: Ever-married females, married only once and below 50 years.

Also married males whose wives had married only once and were below 50 years.

4. Identification and weighting: The sampling frame consisted of 3,870 blocks that were suitably stratified into four strata and arranged according to spatial contiguity within each stratum. Four different samples were selected with probability proportional to size (pps) circular systematically from each stratum with a different random start in each case. From each block households were selected linear systematically.

5. Reponse rate: No information.

B. **Handling of indeterminates**

There are no cases of NAs. However, for some of the questions the responses are indeterminate. For instance, a question for which there can be an indeterminate response is "Do you desire to have more children?" (Yes–1, *Indifferent*–2, No–3). The indeterminate answers have been excluded from all tables except those with percentage distributions.

C. **Prevalence of induced abortion**

This information was obtained in the survey, but specifics are not yet available.

D. **Prevalence of divorce and remarriage**

No information.

E. **Other remarks**

The data have been subjected to scrutiny on the computer with a view to removing discrepancies and inconsistencies. The quality of the data is on the whole satisfactory.

In the tabulations presented, data from only one subsample have been considered. There are four subsamples in all. Each subsample is representative of the population covered by the survey and is expected to give unbiased estimates of the totals.

DELHI

A. Specification of sample

1. Size: The sample for the female survey was 8,230. The number of interviews completed was 7,248.

2. Universe sampled and frame used: The sample chosen for the survey is a household random sample drawn from a universe of households constructed by actual enumeration of a first stage sample of areal blocks, which was in turn drawn from a complete list of blocks, containing 125 to 200 households with a mean around 150 households, into which the entire metropolitan area was divided for the purpose.

3. Primary respondents: The demographic survey comprised a household survey and two complementary male and female fertility surveys. The present tabulation is confined to the female fertility survey. The primary respondent here was an ever-married woman living in the sample household, married only once and below age 50 years. The complementary male survey collected data from ever-married males in the sample household, married only once and below age 55 years. We have, therefore, complementary information collected from husbands of a substantial number of women covered in the female fertility survey.

4. Identification and weighting: There were in all 4,501 areal blocks into which metropolitan Delhi was divided. These were grouped into eight strata, seven of which were individually well-defined zones of local administration and the remaining comprised all blocks selected from different zones for their preponderance of Muslim residence. In effect, we have one stratum comprising predominantly Muslim households and seven strata with almost wholly non-Muslim populations. The first stage sample of blocks was selected by applying a uniform sample fraction of 10 percent in the seven non-Muslim strata and one of 20 percent in the smallest Muslim stratum. The selected sample blocks were completely enumerated in order to construct the universe for drawing the sample of households. The sampling unit is thus the household. In final selection of the households to be included in the universe, we had applied an eligibility criterion as required by the focus of inquiry, namely, fertility behavior. Accordingly, after enumeration, these households that did not have any eligible male or female member were excluded. From the list so compiled for each stratum a random sample of 15 percent was selected.

5. Response rate: The response rate is 88 percent. Among the sample for which interviews could not be completed, we have only 68 cases of refusal; for the remaining bulk of respondents, the schedules could not be completed for a variety of reasons such as inability to contact them even after repeated visits, inability to trace them in cases where they had shifted their residence, and inability to contact them because they had remained out of station during the survey period.

B. Handling of indeterminates

In computation of means and other statistics, the NAs have been excluded. For tables showing percentage distribution they have, however, been included.

C. Prevalence of induced abortion

1.3 percent of pregnancies resulted in induced abortions.

D. Prevalence of divorce and remarriage

By definition, we have covered only women married only once, and so the question of prevalence of remarriage does not arise. Only about 3 percent were either widows or separated and therefore not leading a married life at the time of the survey.

E. Other remarks

In considering these data, it may be worthwhile to note that the population surveyed forms a rather special category in the country's population. It is a metropolitan population and, as such, exhibits a cosmopolitan character. The metropolis, besides being the hub of government activity, is also an important commercial and industrial center of northern India. It enjoys probably the highest level of education and of per capita income in the country. It is further notable that a vigorous family planning program has operated here for more than a decade and a half. Not only do people in general know about family planning, but also they are familiar with the services provided by the government.

RURAL EAST JAVA

A. Specification of sample

1. Size: The sample size of the rural stratum was 2,004, comprising women aged 15–49 years. Only those aged 20–39 years were selected for the comparative study. (1,418 households.)

2. Universe sampled and frame used: The universe comprised 67,977 households, which were stratified into urban (27,052) and rural (40,925), which were situated within areas of five kilometers' radius from three health centers in East Java and one health center in the Municipality of Surabaya. For the comparative study only the rural sample was taken into consideration.

The households were sampled by systematic random selection of census blocks in the respective areas in the first phase, and in the second phase the same method of selection was applied in the sampling of households out of the selected blocks. The sampling frame was then a stratified multistage random selection of households in a selected area in East Java.

3. Primary respondents: The primary respondents were ever-married women aged 15–49 years, and data from those aged 20–39 years were selected for the comparative study. Their husbands were not covered.

4. Identification and weighting: This was an equal probability sample. No weighting was necessary since for the rural stratum the same sample fraction (1/15) was introduced. For urban-rural comparison, however, weighting of samples would be necessary.

5. Response rate: The response rate was 98.4 percent. The proportion of eligible couples interviewed was 99.8 percent.

B. Handling of indeterminates

The NAs are excluded in the calculation of means and percentages, but included in the percentage distributions. For "percent who want no more and are not using contraception," NAs are included in the denominator.

C. Prevalence of induced abortion

The prevalence of induced abortion was not very clear. From the interview, we were able to discover 205 cases with a history of abortion among 2,004 respondents.

D. Prevalence of divorce and remarriage

The incidence of divorce and remarriage was high among the respondents. Among currently married respondents, 19.1 percent had been married twice, 7.5 percent three times, and 4.1 percent four or more times. Among those respondents, 3.2 percent had been divorced once, 1.5 percent had been divorced two or more times.

E. Other remarks

In our study, a substantial portion of respondents gave indeterminate answers to specific questions, which limits the possibility of including them in the comparative analysis. We are still not convinced that most of the women respondents in Indonesia do not have an opinion on matters relating to their fertility behavior.

GREAT BRITAIN

A. Specification of sample

1. Size: Altogether, 2,262 completed interviews were obtained. The weighted "number of cases" arising from these interviews is 2,309. The weighted "number of cases" considered here is 1,088.

2. *Universe sampled and frame used:* The sample was of women living in England and Wales, and Scotland south of the Caledonian Canal. The sampling frame used was the system of electoral registers.

3. *Primary respondents:* The sample design was such that the electoral registers sometimes provided the names of particular individuals, and sometimes the locations of households. Women were interviewed if (1) they had been born in the United Kingdom; (2) they had been born in the year 1907 or later; (3) they had married, and by age 45; (4) they were still married to their first husband at the time of survey, or, if not, had remained married to their first husband until at least age 45; and (5) their first husband had been born in the United Kingdom. Only a part of this sample is considered here, however—namely, those women born in the period 1928–1947, inclusive. (It should be noted that all of these women must still be married to their first husband.)

4. *Identification and weighting:* The sample design involved, first, the selection of a number of parliamentary constituencies (with pps), then the selection of a ward within each of these constituencies (also with pps), and, finally, the selection of fixed numbers of names, and of households, from each of the chosen wards. It should be noted that this procedure necessitated a certain (small) amount of weighting, and that some of the required weights were not whole numbers.

5. *Response rate:* The response rate was of the order of 90 percent.

B. Handling of indeterminates

NAs and indeterminates were excluded from all calculations of means and percentages.

C. Prevalence of induced abortion

No information on the prevalence of induced abortion is available from the survey itself. Nor are there acceptable data for the period prior to the survey from any other source. It is commonly supposed, however, that the incidence of induced abortion may well have been fairly high during this period.

D. Prevalence of divorce and remarriage

The sample women included in the tables are all still married to their first husband.

E. Other remarks

There is relatively little nonstatement in connection with most items. But the nonstatement associated with the "expect more"/"do not expect more" categorization is really quite high (approximately 18 percent), and this affects a substantial proportion of the data presented.

HUNGARY

A. Specification of sample

1. *Size:* 8,800 women, 5,937 of whom were aged 20–39.

2. *Universe sampled and frame used:* The aim was to ensure national representativity to the greatest possible extent. Selection was made in two stages: in the first stage the settlements to be included in the sample were indicated, and in the second stage the dwellings to be enumerated were indicated. The selection of the settlements was performed with stratification.

3. *Primary respondents:* These were married women aged 20–39 years. The sample represents well the Hungarian married female population, presumably not only with respect to age—this is confirmed by the comparison of this criterion with countrywide data—but also to other criteria.

4. *Identification and weighting:* No information.

5. *Response rate:* In the study 0.8 percent refused to give a reply, which —as far as we know—is a very low ratio on an international scale, too. Its contribution to the bias of the sample can be neglected.

B. Handling of indeterminates

NAs were not indicated separately in the tables. At the counting they were not taken into consideration, so the percentage distributions as well as the mean values refer to those responding.

C. Prevalence of induced abortion

In Hungary the very high number of induced abortions exerts a great influence on the "want no more but not using contraception" behavior. In 1972 in Hungary 178,000 induced abortions were carried out, which means 117 induced abortions per 100 live births and 66 induced abortions per 1,000 women aged 15–49 years.

D. Prevalence of divorce and remarriage

The Hungarian study only referred to women living in marriage at the date of interviewing, so divorced women were not interviewed.

It was not the aim of the survey to study the question of divorce and remarriage, so we do not know what percent of the women live in second or third marriages.

INDIA

A. Specification of sample

1. *Size:* In all, 26,054 respondents were interviewed for the family planning survey. This included roughly half males and half females. Out of these, 10,246 females in the age group of 20–39 years were included for analysis carried out for the IUSSP Subcommittee.

2. Universe sampled and frame used: The sampling was designed to be representative of all married couples in India, with wives aged 15–44 years, excepting those living in Jammu and Kashmir, the Northeast Frontier Agency (NEFA), and other offshore territories like Andaman and Nicobars. A multistage stratified sampling design was adopted in the survey. India was first stratified into 14 primary strata comprising political states or groups of states. Each of the primary strata was again stratified into secondary strata—urban and rural areas as defined in the 1961 census of population.

In each state the cities and towns in urban areas were further divided into five strata on the basis of population size as of the 1961 census. In each of the urban substrata thus formed, the sample was selected by using a three-stage sampling procedure. In the first stage the towns were selected with probability proportional to the total population of the sampled towns. In the second stage the dwelling units within each selected town were selected with the help of electoral rolls, by using the systematic sampling procedure with a random start. A selected elector together with his address identified a dwelling unit that was selected. At each of the selected dwelling units, all residents were enumerated. From among those the married members who qualified for interview were identified, and one of them was selected at random for the purpose of interview.

In each state the villages were divided into three strata according to their population size. Villages from stratum one were selected with probability proportional to total size of selected villages. For representing the remaining villages in the state, first a sample of two or more districts was selected, and then from each selected district, two *taluks/tehsils* (subdistricts) were selected. Villages from the selected *taluks/tehsils* were stratified into two strata, and from each of them the required number of villages were selected. The districts, *taluks/tehsils*, and villages were selected on the basis of probability proportional to the total rural population of the sampled units. The procedures adopted in selection of dwelling units and respondents were the same as those used in the case of urban areas. Allocation of sample size of the towns and villages selected within a stratum had been made, as far as possible, in proportion to their population. In all, 261 towns and 722 villages were selected. The sampling fractions for each stratum are given below:

Stratum	*Sampling Fraction*
Towns with population of at least 50,000	25 per 100,000 population
Towns below 50,000 population	20 per 100,000 population
Villages with population of 5,000 and above	10 per 100,000 population
Villages below 5,000 population	3 per 100,000 population

3. Primary respondents: Currently married women aged 15–44 years and currently married men whose wives were aged 15–44 years.

4. Identification and weighting: Each respondent was assigned a weight inversely proportional to the probability of selection.

5. Response rate: No information given.

B. Handling of indeterminates
No information given.

C. Prevalence of induced abortion
No information collected.

D. Prevalence of divorce and remarriage
No information collected.

E. Other remarks
Presumably, the prevalence of induced abortion and divorce and remarriage is too low to significantly affect the results of the survey.

JAKARTA

A. Specification of sample

1. Size: 2,246 households—1,117 males, 1,129 females.

2. Universe sampled and frame used: Jakarta Raya, stratified into two stages. The frame was an administrative scheme. Excluded area: the Seribu Islands (a group of islands in the bay of Jakarta).

3. Primary respondents: Women aged 15–49 and ever married. Husbands not covered.

4. Identification and weighting:

Total number of primary sampling units: 17,174—Sample 1/54 from the whole.

(1/54 × 17,174)

Number of secondary sampling units per primary unit = 40 or 50 households — Sample 1/5

(1/5 × 40 or 50)

5. Response rate: 325 substitutions—approximately 14 percent of the total sample. Specifically:

A. Not Eligible		B. Others	
Too old	89	Could not locate	126
Not married	7	Seriously ill	4
Moved away	72	Others	5
No such person	19		
Dead	3		
	190		135

B. Handling of indeterminates
NAs were not included in calculations of means. This holds for all tables.

C. Prevalence of induced abortion

There were some questions on abortion, but no data are available.

D. Prevalence of divorce and remarriage

There were some questions related to the prevalence of divorce and remarriage, but no tabulation has been made.

E. Other remarks

1. This survey was carried out before the launching of the National Family Planning Program.

2. Reporting of births seems to be exaggerated. This produces high estimates of the level of fertility and crude birth rate.

KOREA

A. Specification of sample

1. Size: Approximately 2,975 dwelling units were sampled; 1,883 women were interviewed.

2. Universe sampled and frame used: A stratified multistage sampling technique was employed to obtain a probability sample. The entire country (excluding offshore islands) was divided into the following five strata, considering the population size and economic characteristics of the local administrative unit:

- A. Seoul—the entire city of Seoul.
- B. Industrial cities—the cities with at least 50,000 persons engaged in manufacturing industry, excluding Seoul. The following nine cities belonged to this stratum: Pusan, Inchon, Suwon, Taejon, Kunsan, Kwangju, Taegu, Masan, and Ulsan.
- C. Small cities—all cities (population 50,000 or more) other than those included in strata A and B and the island city of Cheju. There were 21 cities in this stratum.
- D. Small towns—88 *Eups* (small towns) in the nation, excluding 3 *Eups* on Cheju island.
- E. Rural villages—all *Myuns* (rural villages), excluding those in remote islands.

3. Primary respondents: Primary respondents were all currently married women aged 15–44 years. Interviews were conducted in the respondents' homes.

4. Identification and weighting: Data are weighted when the five strata are combined into national figures.

5. Response rate: 81 percent from a de jure perspective and 91 percent from a de facto perspective.

B. Handling of indeterminates

1. NA (not applicable) responses were excluded (in both numerator and denominator) from the computations of both percentages and means.

2. NR (no response) responses were excluded (in both numerator and denominator) from calculations of the mean. In calculating percentages, NR responses were included in the denominator but not in the numerator.

C. Prevalence of induced abortion

Approximately 20 percent of the Korean women aged 20–39 in the sample had experienced at least one induced abortion. The highest proportions of women having at least one induced abortion were in Seoul and other cities, and the lowest in rural areas.

D. Prevalence of divorce and remarriage

There is no direct evidence from the survey on this issue. Divorce and remarriage, however, are relatively rare in Korea.

E. Other remarks

The 1971 Korea survey is described in more detail in Bom Mo Chung, James A. Palmore, Sang Joo Lee, and Sung Jin Lee, *Psychological Perspectives: Family Planning in Korea* (Seoul, Korea: Hollym Corp. Publishers, 1972).

WEST MALAYSIA, 1966–1967

A. Specification of sample

1. Size: 5,457 women were interviewed.

2. Universe sampled and frame used: The West Malaysian Family Survey was based on a probability sample of all noninstitutional households in West Malaysia. The sample for the survey was divided into three major strata:

  A. Each of the five metropolitan areas (population of 75,000 or more in the 1957 census).

  B. The smaller urban areas (population of 7,660–74,999 in the 1957 census).

  C. The rural areas (population less than 7,660 in the 1957 census).

Further stratification was carried out within the metropolitan areas, so that each of the five metropolitan areas in West Malaysia was represented by an approximately equal number of cases in the sample. All in all, then, there were seven strata: one for each metropolitan area, a small town stratum, and a rural stratum.

3. Primary respondents: Primary respondents were all currently married women 15–44 years of age. All interviews were conducted in the respondents' homes.

4. Identification and weighting: The use of a stratified sampling design requires that the data be weighted when the strata are combined to provide estimates for West Malaysia as a whole.

5. Response rate: 94 percent.

B. Handling of indeterminates

1. NA (not applicable) responses were excluded (in both numerator and denominator) from computations of both percentages and means.

2. NR (no response) responses were excluded (in both numerator and denominator) from calculations of the mean. In calculating percentages, NR responses were included in the denominator but not in the numerator.

C. Prevalence of induced abortion

The prevalence of induced abortion was undoubtedly underreported in the survey. Only 1 percent of the survey respondents reported one or more induced abortions. The actual prevalence is higher; however, the true figures are not known.

D. Prevalence of divorce and remarriage

Eighteen percent of the currently married women aged 15–44 years had been married more than once. Data on marriage are reported in detail in James A. Palmore and Ariffin bin Marzuki, "Marriage patterns and cumulative fertility in West Malaysia: 1966–1967," *Demography* 6, no. 4 (1969):383–401.

E. Other remarks

The Malaysian National Family Planning Board began its program of service activities in May 1967. From October 1966 to April 1967 a baseline survey was carried out by the Malaysian Department of Statistics under the auspices of the Board. This survey was designed to obtain information from an area probability sample of all noninstitutional households in West Malaysia, stressing information on fertility and on family planning knowledge, attitudes, and practices. (The study was confined to West Malaysia because the Board did not intend to begin services in Sabah and Sarawak until some years later.) The survey methodology and selected results have been summarized previously in numerous articles as well as in the book, National Family Planning Board of Malaysia, *Report on the West Malaysian Family Survey, 1966–1967*, Government of Malaysia, Kuala Lumpur, 1968, 534 pp. (prepared by James A. Palmore with the assistance of A. Schnaiberg, C. M. Langford, and D. Fernandez).

WEST MALAYSIA, 1970

A. Specification of sample

1. Size: Approximately 28,000 households and about 44,000 respondents.

2. Universe sampled and frame used: Since the Post-Enumeration Survey was designed primarily as a check of coverage of enumeration by the 1970 Census of Population and Housing, the sample frame used for selection of primary sampling units was the 15,594 Census Enumeration Blocks (EBs), which ranged in size from about 60 to 80 households. The EBs were divided into three separate strata (metropolitan towns, towns, and rural areas) and five geographical regions (south: Johore and Malacca; central: Selangor and Negri Sembilan; northwest: Perak; north: Penang, Kedah, and Perlis; and east: Kelantan, Trengganu, and Pahang).

A sample of 1,138 EBs was selected with probability proportional to size. The census house-listing books provided the frame for selection of households. After renumbering households listed in the census listing books serially from 1, a systematic random sample of about 28,000 households was selected for interview.

3. Primary respondents: There were three categories of respondents: heads of households (male or female), currently married females aged 15–44 years, and ever-married females aged 15–44 years but not currently married. Those interviewed were a total of 25,654 heads of households (including 1,712 ever-married females) and 18,639 ever-married females (of whom 13,449 were currently married). Husbands who were classified as heads of households were interviewed on KAP questions; however, in cases where married males did not happen to be head of the household, they were not interviewed on KAP questions.

4. Identification and weighting: The sample is self-weighting, with selection of primary sampling units (Census Enumeration Blocks) on the basis of probability proportional to size.

5. Response rate: Data not currently available on response rates for categories of respondents.

B. Handling of indeterminates

For all calculations of means in the tables, indeterminate cases were omitted. For example, in the table with mean desired number of sons by wife's age and education 11 percent were excluded, and in the similar table with desired number of children 7 percent were excluded. For distributions, the percentages of indeterminate cases are shown in the relevant tables.

C. Prevalence of induced abortion

No data available from this survey.

D. Prevalence of divorce and remarriage

No data available from this survey.

MEXICO CITY

A. Specification of sample

1. Size: 798 households.

2. Universe sampled and frame used: The data are drawn from a probability sample of households that make up the rough equivalent of the Mexico City urbanized area. This area includes all of the Federal District with the exception of portions of the southern *delegaciones,* which are rural in character, but it also includes parts of the adjacent *municipios* of Atenco, Ecatepec, Naucalpan, Netzahuacoyotl, Tlalnepantla, and Zaragoza. The exclusions amount to about 27,000 dwelling units, whereas the adjacent *municipios* generated an additional quarter million dwelling units for the frame. No block estimates were available for the area, so a double-sampling procedure was employed, involving the listing of over 600 blocks in the first stage and a subselection of over 200 blocks on which interviews were taken. The sample is stratified and clustered in groups of five interviews per block.

3. Primary respondents: Eligible respondents were wives in households containing a married couple.

4. Identification and weighting: The design was not self-weighting, so weights have been employed in the analysis. If more than one couple lived in the household, a printed random selection on the schedule determined which wife was to be interviewed.

5. Response rate: Interviews were completed in 96 percent of the eligible households.

B. Handling of indeterminates

Interviewers were sent back to the households if questions were skipped or missed. At several places in the interview where we anticipated some resistance or ambiguity of response (for example, expected number of additional children), a series of probes written into the schedule were used to convert initially ambiguous responses to numerical responses. The latter were used in all the tables presented. For the remaining one or two percent NAs, random, or internal consistency procedures were used, depending on the particular question involved. In the data presented here, the small number of NAs were eliminated completely. Given the small number of NAs, any procedure used could not have affected the overall results.

C. Prevalence of induced abortion

After obtaining a live birth history, the respondent was asked: "Did you ever have any pregnancies that did not result in a live birth? For instance, stillbirths, miscarriages, or abortions. How many? How did the (1st, 2nd, etc.)

pregnancy end? Was it a stillbirth, miscarriage, or abortion?" About 4 percent of the women reported having had an abortion.

D. Prevalence of divorce and remarriage

About 6 percent of the women reported more than one marriage.

NETHERLANDS

A. Specification of sample

1. Size: 3,000 women.

2. Universe sampled and frame used: The sample consisted of 1,000 women each, from three marriage cohorts of 1958, 1963, and 1968. The sample was taken from 67 municipalities, including all the major cities. All provinces were included.

3. Primary respondents: Married women from the three marriage cohorts, with husband and wife of Dutch nationality. Only first marriages were included, with the marriages still extant at the period of investigation (April–May 1969). Husbands were not covered.

4. Identification and weighting: The number of interviews depended on the size of the municipality, with a minimum of 12 interviews per cohort. No other weighting took place.

5. Response rate: The response rate was 83 percent. Nine percent refused, and 8 percent could not be reached because of change of address or other problem.

B. Handling of indeterminates

NAs have not been included as separate categories or columns in tables, except when explicitly stated.

C. Prevalence of induced abortion

Questions on prevalence of abortion have not been asked.

D. Prevalence of divorce and remarriage

Divorce and remarriage were excluded from our sample, which included first marriages only (see A.3).

E. Other remarks

No special remarks. It is realized that the marriage-cohort approach limits the comparability of these data.

PHILIPPINES

A. Specification of sample

1. Size: 7,237 households consisting of 8,175 ever-married women, 4,788 of them from urban areas; 3,387 from rural areas.

2. Universe sampled and frame used: National frame used—list of households in selected sample areas.

Urban: A simple, stratified two-stage sampling. The first-stage unit was the electoral precinct, and the second-stage unit was the household.

Rural: An almost simple, stratified two-stage sampling was employed. The *barrios* (villages), the first-stage unit, were selected with probability proportional to size of population; the households, the second-stage unit, were selected systematically with a random start.

3. Primary respondents: All ever-married women, 15 years old and over; questions were asked regarding the husband, which could be answered by the ever-married woman.

4. Identification and weighting:
Weighting: urban respondents × 4
rural respondents × 12
Probability proportional to size—rural area
Equal probability sampling—urban area

5. Response rate: No information from this survey.

B. Handling of indeterminates

NRs not included in the calculation of means. (NRs amounted to 3 percent on the question concerning ideal number of sons.)

C. Prevalence of induced abortion

15.9 percent of all marriages reported at least one stillbirth or abortion.

D. Prevalence of divorce and remarriage

3.4 percent of wives and 5.0 percent of husbands were married more than once.

TAIWAN

A. Specification of sample

1967 survey:

1. Size: 4,989.

2. Universe sampled and frame used: The study had a stratified, multistage, cluster probability sample. Excluded were 30 townships with largely aboriginal populations.

3. Primary respondents: Currently married women aged 20–44 years.

4. Identification and weighting: The sample was made to be self-weighting, and probability of selection was proportional to size of stage unit.

5. Response rate: 85 percent. Most noninterviews were the result of failure to locate couples selected from the Household Register or couples who had moved.

1970 survey:

1. Size: 2,689.

2. Universe sampled and frame used: The study was a reinterview of a randomly selected subsample of the women interviewed in 1967, with a supplementary sample of about 405 women aged 22–41 who were married for the first time between October 1967 and October 1969.

3. Primary respondents: Currently married women aged 22–46. A survey of the husbands of most of these women was done in 1969.

4. Identification and weighting: Women aged 18–24 at the time of the 1967 survey were weighted to accurately represent younger women in 1970.

5. Response rate: About 92 percent.

B. Handling of indeterminates

NAs were few (about 1 percent) and were included in distributions, but excluded from the numerators and denominators for calculation of means.

C. Prevalence of induced abortion

12.3 percent of the 1967 sample had had at least one abortion.

D. Prevalence of divorce and remarriage

98 percent of the 1967 sample were in their first marriage.

THAILAND

A. Specification of sample

The data used in this study are based on information recorded in the national sampling survey entitled the Longitudinal Study of Social, Economic and Demographic Change in Thailand, carried out by the Institute of Population Studies of Chulalongkorn University. A national sample of rural households was interviewed in 1969, and a year later a national sample of urban households was interviewed.

1969 RURAL SAMPLE:

1. Size: Almost 1,500 households.

2. Universe sampled and frame used: Some districts were excluded from the sampling universe because they were either predominantly Muslim (those comprise four provinces in the south of Thailand where a specially designed survey is required), too remote to allow one-day return-trip travel from district headquarters by interview teams and still allow time for interviewing, or too politically sensitive to accommodate this type of scientific research. The population of the excluded areas constituted about 18 percent of Thailand's total rural population according to the 1960 census.

3. Primary respondents: Whenever possible and appropriate the male household head, his wife, and all other ever-married women under age 60 living in the household were interviewed. Two interview schedules were used, one for the household head (whether male or female) and the other for ever-married women (including the head of household's wife).

4. Identification and weighting: Selection of households from the non-excluded districts was made through a stratified, three-stage cluster sampling procedure. The stratifying variable was the percentage of population in each district not engaged in agriculture.

5. Response rate: No information available.

1970 URBAN SAMPLE:

1. Size: About 200 households were interviewed in the urban round of this study.

2. Universe sampled and frame used: The population living in the areas legally designated as municipal areas was considered to constitute the urban population. Municipal areas that were located in the predominantly Muslim provinces or that lacked a safe route to reach them were excluded from the sampling universe. The excluded municipal areas comprised a little less than 5 percent of Thailand's total urban population according to the 1960 census.

3. Primary respondents: Presumably, the same as for the rural sample.

4. Identification and weighting: Selection of households in the nonexcluded municipal areas was again made through a stratified, three-stage cluster sampling procedure proportional to size, although for the urban sample the stratification was on the basis of regional location, with the Bangkok metropolitan area constituting a separate stratum.

5. Response rate: No information available.

B. Handling of indeterminates

NAs were excluded from the means, but included in distributions. NAs amounted to around 15–18 percent on the question concerning ideal number of children.

C. Prevalence of induced abortion

No information available.

D. Prevalence of divorce and remarriage

No information available.

UNITED STATES

A. Specification of sample
1965 study:
1. Size: 5,617.

2. *Universe sampled and frame used:* National area.

3. *Primary respondents:* Currently married women under age 55, residing in the coterminous United States and able to participate in an English language interview.

4. *Identification and weighting:* Probability sample.

5. *Response rate:* No information.

1970 study:

1. *Size:* 6,752.

2. *Universe sampled and frame used:* National area.

3. *Primary respondents:* Ever-married women under age 45, residing in the coterminous United States and able to participate in an English language interview.

4. *Identification and weighting:* Probability sample.

5. *Response rate:* No information.

B. Handling of indeterminates

In all tables, the relatively few respondents with missing data (DK or NA) on any variable included in the table are excluded from both the calculation of the statistic and the reported Ns.

C. Prevalence of induced abortion

For the women in the sample this is unknown. However, national statistics from the Center for Disease Control indicate that at the time of the study abortion was primarily used by never-married women and formerly married women, rather than currently married women.

D. Prevalence of divorce and remarriage

The marital history of all ever-married women in the 1970 sample is as follows:

	Percent
Currently married, once married	80
Currently married, married more than once	10
Formerly married, once	8
Formerly married, more than once	2
	100

E. Other remarks

Since both the 1965 and 1970 studies double-sampled blacks, a weighting system based on the Current Population Reports was used to estimate parameters for the total population. When reporting the number of respondents upon which a given statistic was based, unweighted numbers were reported.

Soc
HB
891
F73

LUIS

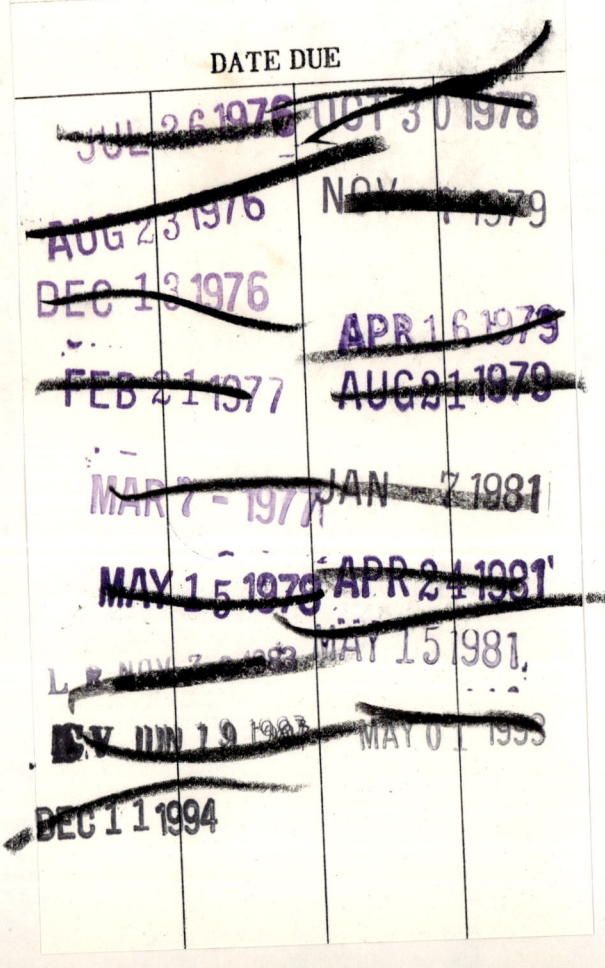